MOSBY'S

TOUR GUIDE
TO NURSING SCHOOL

A Student's Road Survival Kit

In Collaboration with NSNA
National Student Nurses' Association, Inc.

MOSBY'S
TOUR GUIDE TO NURSING SCHOOL

A Student's Road Survival Kit

FIFTH EDITION

MELODIE CHENEVERT, RN, BSN, MN, MA
Pro-Nurse
Gaithersburg, Maryland

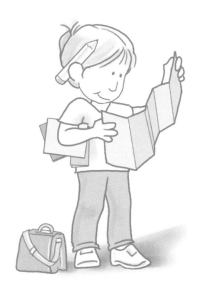

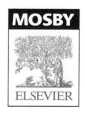

MOSBY

ELSEVIER

MOSBY
ELSEVIER

11830 Westline Industrial Drive
St. Louis, Missouri 63146

Mosby's Tour Guide to Nursing School: ISBN-13: 978-0-323-03763-1
A Student's Road Survival Kit   ISBN-10: 0-323-03763-1

Notice

Neither the Publisher nor the Authors assume any responsibility for any loss or injury and/or damage to persons or property arising out of or related to any use of the material contained in this book. It is the responsibility of the treating practitioner, relying on independent expertise and knowledge of the patient, to determine the best treatment and method of application for the patient.

The Publisher

ISBN-13: 978-0-323-03763-1
ISBN-10: 0-323-03763-1

Senior Editor: *Yvonne Alexopoulos*
Editorial Assistant: *Sarah Vales*
Publishing Services Manager: *Deborah L. Vogel*
Project Manager: *Deon Lee*
Design Manager: *Bill Drone*
Illustrator: *Jeanne Robertson*

Working together to grow
libraries in developing countries

www.elsevier.com | www.bookaid.org | www.sabre.org

ELSEVIER   BOOK AID International   Sabre Foundation

Printed in the United States of America

Last digit is print number: 9 8 7 6 5 4 3

*Dedicated to the future nurse
and
the future of nursing . . .
they are one and the same*

Note to Students

I am very proud that NSNA has collaborated with Melodie Chenevert and Mosby to bring you *Mosby's Tour Guide to Nursing School*. A year into nursing school, I can say with confidence that everything this book says is true! It also covers all the important aspects of nursing school, from grades to clinicals, and presents it all in a highly readable style. Even though I wish I had read this book at the beginning of nursing school, I still found many pieces of advice and bits of information that will help me this year—it's never too late to put the information in this book into practice. This is also the perfect book to use over and over to inspire you, help get you over the rough spots, and just remind you about the important things on your journey.

Nursing school is a whole new ballgame. I came to it after teaching for over a decade and taking time off somewhere in the middle to go to school full time for a Masters in teaching. Needless to say, I felt pretty confident that I knew how to "do" school when I started nursing school. But nursing school is different from liberal arts programs because the coursework is completely cumulative and interrelated. As one of my professors was fond of saying, you can "flush" the material after the test, but it is not in your best interest to do so because you will need to know it for clinicals, other classes, and of course, the NCLEX.

The other unique thing about nursing school is the heavy emphasis on hands-on, experiential learning. So I admit I have found it to be quite a challenge. I look back and am amazed at how far I've come in only one year, but there's no time to rest on my laurels—I still have a long way to go. I think it's like trying to learn a language, a musical instrument, or a sport; practice is the key. That's why many people say the second year is easier than the first—because they've practiced enough and know how to succeed. This book can give you an edge to help you make the first year easier—when you take tests, interact with professors, and go to clinicals.

The NSNA mission involves mentoring nursing students, conveying ethical standards, advocating for high-quality health care, and developing future nursing leaders. This book is meant to mentor, and that alone makes it the perfect tool for NSNA members. However, if you can internalize its messages, I think you will be well on your way to achieving all the other aspects of the NSNA mission.

I love this book because, at heart, it is really all about YOU. Not YOU the nursing student, just plain YOU. The down-to-earth advice presented here can be applied to lots of areas of life, not just to nursing school. The bottom line is to be true to yourself and what you want out of life, and if that is nursing, then so much the better!

Rebecca Wheeler
President
National Student Nurses' Association, Inc.

Foreword

We often hear nursing students say that they did not choose the path of nursing but that nursing chose them. It may well be that nursing's core values are what call us to the field and that our desire to live out these values drives us to the profession. These same core values help us to define nursing and to determine how we navigate our professional journey.

Your journey through nursing school—in the classroom, in clinicals, and as part of a professional organization—is preparation for the real world. In nursing school, values may be challenged and questioned, and sometimes even doubted. When this happens, it is a good time to reflect and see just how deep those values go. Like in life, when we start to doubt our route, it's a good idea to pull out a road map and consult it for directions! This can determine which road—or roads—will best serve you along the way. Remember, don't be discouraged by detours—they will often get you back to the path you're seeking.

On this journey, it is also important to remember that educational and health care institutions have their own road maps and that many are guided by their core values. Matching your value system with that of an employer may very well be what makes the difference between accepting a job offer at hospital A or driving across town to work in hospital B. An organization's mission, vision, and core values should be plainly visible and incorporated into all aspects of patient care. Think of these values as the landmarks you'll use to make sure you are staying on the road of your choice. Values such as integrity, respect, diversity, collaboration, advocacy, holism, and social justice, among others, are idle words unless they are practiced. They should be considered with every decision and with every turn that you take down the road.

Your journey into the profession of nursing is just beginning. You have found your way into one of the most rewarding and respected professions a person can wish for. Now that nursing has chosen you—and you have followed your heart and sharpened your intellect—enjoy the journey and don't forget your tour guide!

Diane J. Mancino, EdD, RN, CAE
Executive Director
National Student Nurses' Association, Inc.

Preface

ARE YOU MAN ENOUGH TO BE A NURSE? WELL, ARE YOU?

These words were emblazoned on the hottest selling T-shirt at the National Student Nurses' Association convention. I bought the last one. It was way too big for me, but I couldn't resist. It made me smile.

It reminded me of the time I spoke in Houston at a city-wide extravaganza honoring graduating nursing students. A young man glanced at my name tag. "You!" he exclaimed. "You're the person who wrote that book! You're the person who got me through nursing school!" He grabbed me and gave me a big hug. It was a wonderful moment. I have never been more proud of being the author of *Mosby's Tour Guide to Nursing School*. It's a book that has helped many people—men and women—get through nursing school, and it can help you too.

You are holding the fifth edition. Everything has been updated. Here's the information you need on everything from boosting your test scores to boosting your self-esteem, from conducting a study group to overcoming procrastination, from choosing electives to improving term papers to avoiding collisions between your personal and professional lives. Plus you will find candid comments, examples, and ideas from other nursing students.

You have picked a great time to enter nursing school. Scholarships, loans, and grants are readily available. Nurses are in big demand. Salaries are skyrocketing. All the old, cranky nurses are tired. They will be thrilled to see fresh new faces. They know if they don't help you become an excellent nurse, there won't be anyone to take care of them.

One outstanding feature of this survival guide is that it tackles the challenges faced by a "mature" student. Nursing educators used to call anyone older than 20 and other than female a "nontraditional" student. Today female students under 20 are the exception, not the rule. Although typical nursing students are still overwhelmingly female, men are also finding rewarding careers in nursing. Nursing students are older and wiser and much more encumbered than they used to be. Students bring a lot of baggage—obligations, responsibilities, commitments, constraints, and conflicts—all of which make being a successful student much more challenging.

Although this book is primarily designed for the "first-time travelers," nurses returning for advanced degrees and experienced students from other fields making a career switch into nursing have reported the strategies and suggestions in the *Tour Guide* most helpful.

So grab a copy of this book and come on along. You are about to embark on a great journey. Destination: NURSING. It's a rough trip but worth every mile.

Most travelers on this route have a lot in common. Most of us are practical idealists. You know—the sort of people who want to save the human race but who also know the value of a regular paycheck.

As a practical idealist myself, I know it's not easy keeping your feet on the ground while your head is in the clouds. Nursing is one of the few professions that enables you to make such a long stretch.

Nursing is practically ideal. Not only will you earn a good living, you will help others in the process. You will have the knowledge and skills to convert your good intentions into good actions. Although you will not be able to save the whole planet, occasionally you will save one of its occupants. That will be enough. And you will be paid for your services, although perhaps not as much as your skill will deserve.

Nursing school can make you wise beyond your years, but it sometimes also makes you old before your time. This tour guide/survival kit will help you achieve more in nursing school with less wear and tear on your body, mind, and spirit.

Too many "sky's-the-limit" students trip over their own shoelaces, so this book is designed to make sure you don't lose your footing or your ideals. Its down-to-earth tips can help make an average student good and a good student great.

From the beginning this book has been a collaborative effort. Not only has it involved Mosby, the National Student Nurses' Association, and me, it reflects input from countless students and nurses throughout the United States and Canada.

There is only one person who can make this book any better: YOU! Your input can make sure this tour guide/survival kit keeps doing the job it was designed to do—help nursing students survive and even thrive.

If you would like to make a suggestion, share an experience, give a recommendation, or pass along a hot tip, write to me. I promise to respond.

Bon voyage!

Melodie Chenevert, RN, BSN, MN, MA
c/o Nursing Division, Elsevier Inc.
11830 Westline Industrial Drive
St. Louis, MO 63146

"It is a rough road that leads to the heights of greatness."

SENECA

Contents

1 TICKET TO RIDE, 2
Nursing is more than a great living. It's a great life. Career options to last a lifetime.

2 THE STARTING LINEUP, 10
If you've been admitted to a school of nursing, you can do anything! Cooperation, not competition, will bring success.

3 IS THIS TRIP REALLY NECESSARY?, 12
Determining whether you have what it takes to be a nurse. Diverse demands on a working nurse.

4 DESTINATION: REGISTERED NURSE, 20
Tangible and intangible rewards of nursing.

5 HOW LONG WILL THIS TRIP TAKE?, 26
Three preparatory paths to nursing. Career aspirations and financial and time considerations determine the length of education.

6 HOW MUCH WILL THIS TRIP COST?, 32
Calculating and defraying expenses. Being a smart consumer and getting your money's worth.

7 RULES OF THE ROAD, 38
Don't fight the system—work with it. Know your school's rules and follow them to the letter. Collisions between personal freedoms and professional responsibilities.

8   SLOWER TRAFFIC KEEP RIGHT, 42
Survival tips from students to students: take care of
yourself, take care of each other, take one day at a
time, and take care of business.

9   DRIVING INSTRUCTORS, 48
The importance of knowing faculty members thoroughly
and understanding the many roles they play.

10   MORE MILES PER GALLON, 54
Time management from A to Z.

11   DETOURS, 64
Turning wishes into goals and goals into
accomplishments. Issues for the student who must
work while going to school.

12   YOU CAN'T GET THERE FROM HERE, 70
Problem-solving and assertiveness skills.

13   DRIVE-UP TELLER, 76
Making the best use of your memory bank: listening
and learning; reading and remembering.

14   TOLLBOOTH, 86
Test-taking skills designed to boost your grades.

15   TOTALED, 96
Dealing with failure: major or minor.

16   HOW TO JUMP-START YOUR BATTERY, 102
Procrastination and motivation.

17   10-4, GOOD BUDDY, 108
How to form and conduct study groups. Supporting
each other.

18   PREVENTIVE MAINTENANCE, 116
The importance of taking care of yourself.

19   SCENIC ROUTES, 120
Choosing electives.

20   ALTERNATIVE ROUTES, 124
Diversity within the nursing profession. Increasing tolerance and flexibility. How to keep judgmental attitudes from interfering with professional performance.

21   BUSINESS ROUTES, 128
Improving oral and written reports.

22   HOT-WIRED, 138
Internet for nurses.

23   IN THE DRIVER'S SEAT, 150
Taking full responsibility for your actions.

24   SHIFTING GEARS, 152
Difficulties of being a spouse/parent/student. Challenges of returning to school after a long absence. Making the transition from person to professional.

25   MOVING VIOLATIONS, 164
Making the most of the nursing skills lab. Getting adequate experience in the clinical setting.

26   DEFENSIVE DRIVING, 170
Rights and responsibilities. Conforming to the letter or the spirit of the law. Paperwork.

27   STREET SMART, 184
Surviving on tough turf. The importance of first impressions and body language.

28   LIFE IN THE FAST LANE, 190
Last-minute suggestions from senior students.

29   ARE WE THERE YET?, 194
Transition from experienced student to inexperienced professional. But if you have gotten this far, you can do anything!

APPENDIXES

A   Common Prefixes and Suffixes Used in Nursing, 199
B   Sources of Scholarships and Loans, 205
C   State Nurses Associations, 209
D   Canadian Nurses Associations, 213
E   Specialty Nursing Organizations, 215
F   U.S. State and Territorial Boards of Nursing, 219
G   Resources for NCLEX® Review Available from
     Mosby/Elsevier, 223

MOSBY'S
TOUR GUIDE
TO NURSING SCHOOL
A Student's Road Survival Kit

In Collaboration with NSNA
National Student Nurses' Association, Inc.

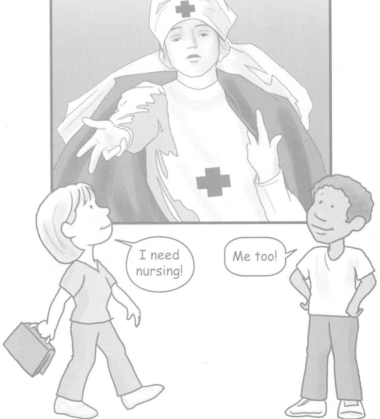

Ticket to Ride

"Finding meaningful, absorbing work is one of the straightest routes to a happier life."
—Anna Quindlen

*D*id you ever stop at a tourist information booth? There are racks full of brochures telling you everything to see and do. The sponsors of these information booths want you to enjoy your visit so much you'll want to live there.

If I were designing a brochure for nursing, it would look something like this:

NURSING

It's more than a good living. It's a good life!

Good living. The average nursing salary is about $48,000 a year. Fringe benefits are excellent. Job security is unparalleled. Because the nurse shortage is a national crisis, generous scholarships and interest-free loans are available for basic and advanced education.

Good life. Nursing is the most portable career you can have. You can literally get a job anywhere in the world. Flexible schedules make it possible to combine a fulfilling family life and a challenging career. You can work in a hospital, clinic, school, home health agency, or industry; you can join the military or create your own business. There are opportunities in education, management, and research. As a nurse you will help people of all ages, incomes, races, religions, and cultures. Yes, becoming a nurse is hard work and being a nurse is a tough job, but every day you will be someone's hero.

Then I'd tell you 101 things you could see and do. For example:

As a new nurse your first job will probably be in a *hospital*. You will be able to choose from dozens of opportunities. In fact, you could spend your entire career in one hospital and never explore all the options.

First, there are so many different clinical specialties. Just name any body part and there is a specialty built around it— eyes, ears, nose, toes, bones, heart, guts, brain. Then choose whether you want to be a *bedside nurse* giving direct patient care, a *specialist*, an *educator*, a *researcher*, a *supervisor*, a *manager*, or an *executive*. There are *admission nurses* and *discharge planning nurses* and nurses who serve as *patient advocates*. You could be an *infection control nurse* or work in *quality assurance*.

You might choose to work in a doctor's *office* or a *clinic*. You might choose *urgent care* where people who don't have a family physician but who don't need an emergency department can go for treatment. You might choose to work in an *emergency department*, become a *trauma nurse specialist*, or a *triage nurse* who sorts patients and prioritizes their needs. You might be the *transport nurse* in the ambulance or the *flight-for-life nurse* on a helicopter.

You might choose *surgery*. There are many different roles for nurses in and around the *operating room*. You might prepare patients for surgery; be the *scrub nurse* or *first assistant* who is literally the doctor's right hand; be a *nurse anesthetist* who puts patients to sleep and monitors them throughout surgery; or be the *postanesthesia nurse* who keeps patients safe until they are awake, alert, and transferred to a regular hospital room.

You might be a *neuroscience nurse* specializing in *brain tumors*, *strokes*, or *spinal cord injuries*. You can provide care when patients are gravely ill or when they are in *rehabilitation* re-learning the basics such as how to walk, talk, read, or eat again.

If you like cutting-edge technology, you can work as a *critical care nurse*. You can be a nurse on the *transplant team.* (We transplant hearts, lungs, livers, kidneys, bone marrow, and more.) *Dialysis nurses* work with patients who are waiting for kidney transplants or who are ineligible for transplants. *Oncology nurses* work with cancer patients. Some become *chemotherapy* or *radiation therapy experts.*

Do you like babies? Then you might work in *labor and delivery* or the *newborn nursery.* You can teach *prenatal classes* for expectant moms and dads. You could become a *nurse midwife* and deliver babies in homes as well as in hospitals. (Nurse midwives in rural areas used to ride horseback. You'll be glad to know that today they drive Jeeps.) You might be a *well-baby nurse specialist* or a *Neonatal Intensive Care Unit (NICU) nurse* helping the tiniest babies survive and thrive. You can be a *lactation consultant* helping mothers be successful at breastfeeding. There are *nurse sonographers* who do ultrasound tests to monitor unborn babies and nurses who specialize in *genetic counseling.*

At the other end of the spectrum, we have *hospice nurses* who help patients and their families in the last stages of life have a dignified, comfortable death. *Palliative care nurses* provide comfort to patients undergoing difficult treatments. They specialize in pain management and symptom control.

Variety is the spice of life for *medical-surgical nurses.* They care for patients in every category. *Orthopedic nurses* specialize in treating patients with bone and joint injuries and disorders. *Cardiac nurses* work with heart patients in all phases of their care. You can work in the *burn unit.*

Gerontology nurses care for the oldest old. *Pediatric nurses* care for children through adolescence. Both do everything a general medical-surgical nurse would do but with a twist. The very young and the very old have special needs during surgery, acute care, and rehabilitation.

You can be a *camp nurse* for kids or run an *adult day care center* for the elderly. You can work in a *nursing home.* You can own a nursing home!

You could become a *public health nurse* and work in the community. You might be a *visiting nurse* who sees people in their homes. You might specialize in the needs of *migrant workers*, join the *Indian Health Service*, or work with the homeless. You could be a *Peace Corps* volunteer, sign on with the *World Health Organization* (WHO), or serve on the *Ship Hope* as it sails the world providing state-of-the-art care to under-served populations. You could become a *cruise ship nurse* and care for the idle rich. *Club Med* and *Disneyland* hire nurses too!

You could become a *medical missionary* and travel to the remote corners of the earth. Or you could become a *parish nurse*, sponsored by your local church to care for its parishioners and reach out to those in need right in your own neighborhood.

If you have an itch to travel, you can sign up with a *traveling nurse agency.* These agencies usually place nurses for 3- to 6-month assignments. All expenses are paid, and traveling nurses may earn twice as much as regular nurses.

School nurses work with students in preschool programs right up through college health clinics. They do some first aid; lots of health screening and physical exams; and even more teaching, counseling, and consulting.

As a *research nurse*, you could work at any university. You might go to Washington, DC, and work at the *National Institutes of Health* (NIH) where nurses are doing procedures that are too new or too intensive for a general hospital or that require much more laboratory and scientific support than it could provide. Or you might go to Atlanta and work for the *Centers for Disease Control and Prevention* (CDC). You might become a *clinical trials project manager* who sets timelines, tracks projects, develops budgets, and secures contracts. You could become a *drug safety monitor.*

You might work for an *insurance company* doing *health screening* and *physical exams.* You can decide which procedures are covered by the policy and whether or not to reimburse hospitals and physicians. You might be an *investigator* and look for fraud.

You might be a *legal nurse consultant* and serve as an *expert witness* in trials. You can become a *nurse attorney.* You can become a *Sexual Assault Nurse Examiner* (SANE) who examines rape victims, preserves evidence, acts as an advocate, and provides counseling. Nurses also work in *prisons* and other correctional facilities.

Nurses serve in the *military*. Where there are troops or battlefields, you will always find nurses. You might work in a *veterans hospital* or even become a *four-star general!*

The *health and fitness industry* hires lots of nurses to help folks do everything from lose weight to stop smoking. *Occupational health nurses* work for small businesses and large corporations. (Healthy employees mean a healthy bottom line.) They do lots of trouble-shooting and preventive health care. They provide *employee-assistance programs* to help people in *crisis* or people with *addictions*.

You can work as a *psychiatric nurse*, helping everyone from autistic children to elders with *Alzheimer's disease*. You can be a *therapist* in *private practice* seeing patients independently or you can work for a *mental health clinic*, *group home*, or *state hospital*. You can answer *crisis hotline* calls, deal with *suicide prevention*, or become a *stress management specialist*.

Teaching is part of every nurse's job, but some nurses specialize in teaching. *Inservice educators* keep the staff informed about new policies, procedures, medications, and equipment. *Patient educators* teach patients and their families about their illnesses, medications, treatments, and options. *Schools of nursing* have *deans*, *professors*, *assistant professors*, *instructors*, *teaching assistants*, *research assistants*, *guest lecturers*, and *clinical faculty*. Clinically speaking, you might become a *diabetes educator* or an *asthma expert*.

You could become a *case manager* who coordinates care for patients with chronic illnesses, making sure treatment is not overdone or left undone.

Clinical nurse specialists are usually experts in one clinical area (heart, lung, maternal-child, cancer). They teach other health care professionals how to give optimum care. They also provide direct care to patients and families as well as coordinate multidisciplinary teams.

Nurse practitioners are super-charged nurses who often substitute for physicians as primary caregivers, perform advanced procedures, and prescribe drugs.

Pharmaceutical companies and hospital equipment manufacturers love to hire nurses as *sales representatives*. Nurses become *consultants* to architectural firms, human resource companies, the motion picture industry, and politicians. Nurses become politicians! Nurses have been elected to the House and the Senate.

Nurses become *authors* and *editors*. Nurses become *inventors* and *entrepreneurs*. There are *nurse ethicists*, *nurse sociologists*, and *nurse anthropologists*. And the list goes on. . . .

It's been said that the average person will have three careers and six to ten jobs in a lifetime. If you become a nurse, you can do that and never leave nursing!

Some of these options require advanced degrees or additional licenses. But many of these just require guts, gumption, persistence, and imagination.

But before you can explore any of these opportunities, you need to go to nursing school. It's your ticket to the ride of a lifetime.

*"There is only one success—to be able to spend your life
in your own way."*
—Christopher Morley

*"We are here on earth to do good for others. What the others
are here for, I don't know."*
—W. H. Auden

*"Time is the coin of your life. It is the only coin you have,
and only you can determine how it will be spent.
Be careful lest you let other people spend it for you."*
—Carl Sandburg

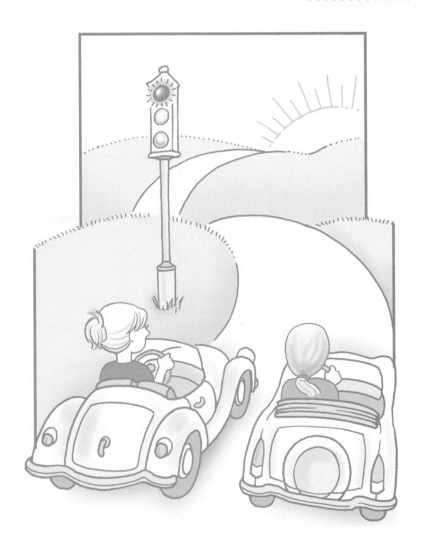

The Starting Lineup

"Nothing great was ever achieved without enthusiasm."
—Ralph Waldo Emerson

*T*he first thing many students do is size up the competition. They think of getting an education as a fiercely competitive race. They jockey for first position as though only one student will be allowed to graduate.

Whether or not you're this competitive, it's only human to look at your classmates and wonder about your comparative status. You may even begin to wonder whether the faculty knew what they were doing when they admitted you. After all, how can they expect you to compete with a fellow who served as a medic in the military, a woman who is old enough to be your mother, a high school valedictorian, and a person who holds a bachelor's degree in psychology?

Relax. You are not expected to *compete* with other students. You are expected to *cooperate* with them.

Instead of a race, think of this educational venture as a caravan about to undertake a long journey. The ultimate goal is to get everyone in your class to the final destination. It is cooperation, not competition, that will bring you success.

Everyone in your class has an excellent chance to graduate because everyone here is already a winner. All have won a place at the starting gate. Considering the rigors of the admission process: getting here was no small accomplishment. If you have managed to get admitted to a school of nursing, YOU CAN DO ANYTHING!

So start your engines. We're off and running.

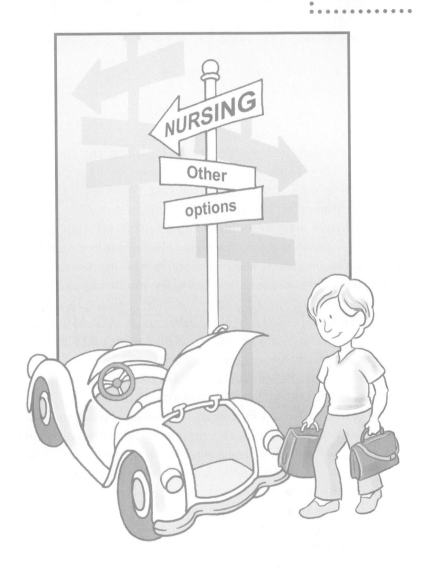

Is This Trip Really Necessary?

"I shall be telling this with a sigh
Somewhere ages and ages hence:
Two roads diverged in a wood,
and I—I took the one less traveled by,
And that has made all the difference."
—Robert Frost, "The Road Not Taken"

*B*efore you begin this long journey, double-check to make sure you know where you are going and what you will find when you get there. If you want to work as a nurse, you are on the right road. If you actually want to work as an airline flight attendant or a health care administrator, you are on the wrong road or, at least, the *long* road. Don't think of nursing education as a "good background" or a "springboard" to another job or profession.

People who choose nursing usually have other interests besides just making a living. They are looking for a way of life that is compatible with their humanitarian instincts.

Will you be successful and happy as a nurse? Answer the following questions. Are you reliable? Do you reach out for responsibility? Are you a good student? Do you have an inquiring mind? Are you adaptable? Do you have a good sense of humor? Are you tolerant? Generous? Discreet? Are you in good health, physically and emotionally?

This list of questions appeared in a two-page advertisement from New York Life Insurance Company published in the *Saturday Evening Post* back in 1955. I happened upon it in an antique store.

New York Life had sponsored a series of advertisements on career opportunities ranging from farming to teaching to engineering. The series was designed to help parents assess which careers might be right for their children. The questions I asked you were the ones parents were to ask themselves about their children before recommending a career in nursing.

At the end of the piece, it said that if you "have the qualities of mind and heart and spirit that nursing demands" you will receive, "in return, rewards far beyond wealth— rewards that never can be lost or stolen: a life of stimulating contacts, honor and respect in your community, and the priceless satisfaction of knowing that every hour of your working life has been of use to others."

Having a relative or a friend with a severe handicap or health problem can be a real source of inspiration. It can also be a real source of guilt. Sometimes people who venture into nursing are on guilt trips. They are trying to make up for things that happened in the past.

WHAT IT IS AND WHAT IT ISN'T

If you think nursing is an insurance policy—something nice to "fall back on" in case you are forced to work at some point in the future—think again. Rapid developments in science and technology make it difficult even for working nurses to keep their skills current.

Nurses who drop out of the profession for a few years have been finding it increasingly difficult, and often impossible, to re-enter nursing. The once-a-nurse-always-a-nurse guarantee may have expired. For example, an Iowa nurse who had been out of the profession for 10 years decided to return to nursing. At every interview she was told that first choice in hiring went to employed nurses seeking transfers, second choice went to new graduates, and third choice went to former nurses who had completed a refresher course. The Catch-22 was that there were no refresher courses being offered in Iowa at that time.

If you think nursing is the road to perpetual job security, think again. For more than 40 years (1942 to the mid-1980s), that was essentially true because the demand for nurses exceeded the supply. By 1984, however, astonished nurses in many parts of the United States suddenly faced layoffs and a very tight job market.

Although analysts saw this "surplus" of nurses as an artificial glitch and predicted the shortage would soon re-appear, the damage was already done. Potential nursing students turned away from the profession in droves. In 1986 schools of nursing reported drops in enrollment of *up to 50%*.

That bad news proved to be good news for nurses and nursing students. As the economy recovered, the demand for nurses skyrocketed. Funding for education increased. Salaries shot up dramatically. Hospitals went to great lengths to attract and keep good nurses.

The nurse shortage made national headlines. Schools of nurses were filled to overflowing. In 1993, for every student admitted to a school of nursing, two students had to be turned away.

But by then the nation's economy was in serious trouble. The early 1990s looked just like the early 1980s. The nurse shortage? What nurse shortage? Hospitals were merging, downsizing, and closing. Suddenly, experienced nurses flooded the market. In many areas of the country, new graduates were hard pressed to find entry-level positions.

Boom. Bust. Boom. Bust.

In the late 1990s, hospitals continued to "dispose" of nurses, hoping to replace them with less expensive personnel. Salaries stagnated, fringe benefits were reduced, and important perks such as flexible schedules disappeared. Nurses entered the new millennium battered and bruised.

Overnight something changed. Suddenly, hospitals were bulging with patients, and there weren't enough nurses to provide care. Actually, it wasn't sudden at all. Our population is aging, and older people just require more care.

Hospitals that had pitched out nurses were now asking their nurses to pitch in—to work double shifts, come in on their days off, and cancel vacations. But the nurses had aged too. Many were not ready, willing, or able to rise to the challenge. I hope you will be able to rise to the challenge.

In 2001 the nurse shortage was again a national crisis. Déjà vu. Enrollment in schools of nursing had declined steadily over the previous 6 years. In one prestigious school of nursing, the number of freshmen entering had dropped from 90 to 25.

Local, state, and federal task forces began working frantically to reverse the trend. Money was pumped into scholarships and interest-free loans. Nurse recruiters, used to attending high school career fairs, found themselves promoting nursing in middle schools, elementary schools, and even preschools!

Johnson & Johnson pumped millions of dollars into a public service advertising campaign to promote nursing as great career. You have probably seen their "Dare to Care" TV ads, posters, and brochures. If you haven't visited their website, you should. It is *http://www.discovernursing.com.*

Health care reform is inevitable, but what that reform will actually entail is anyone's guess. It promises to be an exciting time for nurses.

Today 60% of all nurses work in hospitals. The rest work in other settings—the home, the school, the clinic, the community. You will hear a lot about "advanced practice nurses." These are nurses with graduate degrees who are equipped to provide primary care.

So before you follow the yellow brick road to nursing, you should be sure to separate fact from fantasy. For example, if you think a nurse's primary function is to assist the doctor, you have been watching too much television. In real life nurses spend very little time working alongside doctors. Nurses usually work alone.

WHAT DO NURSES DO ALL DAY?

Nursing is not a do-as-you-are-told job. It is a profession that demands the ability to interview, observe, analyze, detect, develop, write, teach, interpret, counsel, coordinate, collaborate, insert, inject, dispense, change, document, count, order, improvise, supervise, create, give, and take.

In one day you may be called on to do such diverse tasks as interview patients, document progress, develop care plans, write discharge summaries, teach self-care, interpret laboratory findings, insert tubes, check monitors, maintain life-support machinery, counsel grief-stricken families, collaborate with other health care professionals, analyze problems, assess potentials, irrigate wounds, change dressings, collect specimens, coordinate care during birth or death, dispense medications, take temperatures, and give hope.

Much of a nurse's time is spent in direct patient care. Most nurses wish it could be more. Unfortunately, nurses are also saddled with lots of other tasks, such as transcribing doctors' orders, counting narcotics, ordering supplies, directing traffic, enforcing policies, maintaining schedules, answering telephones, delivering dinner trays, cleaning utility rooms, obtaining equipment, running errands, and mopping up messes.

The general-duty, all-purpose, industrial-strength registered nurse must be ready, willing, and able to deliver everything from mail to babies. Obviously, it takes much more than a nice personality, a ready smile, and good intentions to make a good nurse. It takes more substance than fluff to be a successful nurse.

Are you fluff or substance? To find out, take this quiz:

DO YOU HAVE...

1.	A strong background in math and science?	☐ Yes	☐ No
2.	Good hand-eye coordination?	☐ Yes	☐ No
3.	Lots of common sense?	☐ Yes	☐ No
4.	The ability to stay calm in emergencies?	☐ Yes	☐ No
5.	Excellent communication skills?	☐ Yes	☐ No
6.	A sound body?	☐ Yes	☐ No
7.	A stable mind?	☐ Yes	☐ No
8.	An above-average intellect?	☐ Yes	☐ No
9.	An affinity for machines and computers?	☐ Yes	☐ No
10.	A compassionate heart?	☐ Yes	☐ No
11.	Teaching abilities?	☐ Yes	☐ No
12.	Leadership qualities?	☐ Yes	☐ No
13.	Patience, tolerance, flexibility, persistence?	☐ Yes	☐ No
14.	A strong ego?	☐ Yes	☐ No
15.	An affinity for problem solving?	☐ Yes	☐ No
16.	Confidence in your decision-making abilities?	☐ Yes	☐ No
17.	Good organizational skills?	☐ Yes	☐ No
18.	Reliable powers of observation?	☐ Yes	☐ No
19.	The ability to see the best in people in the worst of times?	☐ Yes	☐ No
20.	No objection to working on Christmas?	☐ Yes	☐ No

FILL IN ONE BLOCK FOR EVERY "YES" ANSWER

FLUFF   **SUBSTANCE**

☐ ☐ ☐ ☐ ☐ ☐ ☐ ☐ ☐ ☐ ☐ ☐ ☐ ☐ ☐ ☐ ☐ ☐ ☐ ☐

If you have all of the qualities outlined in the quiz, skip nursing and go directly to sainthood. You are not only too good for nursing, you are too good to be true. But the more of these attributes you have, the more likely you are to make a success of nursing—and the more likely nursing is to make a success of you.

*"Opportunities are usually disguised as hard work,
so most people don't recognize them."*
—Ann Landers

*"Advice is what we ask for when we already know the answer
but wish we didn't."*
—Erica Jong

"Never mistake motion for action."
—Ernest Hemingway

"Tact is the knack of making a point without making an enemy."
—Sir Isaac Newton

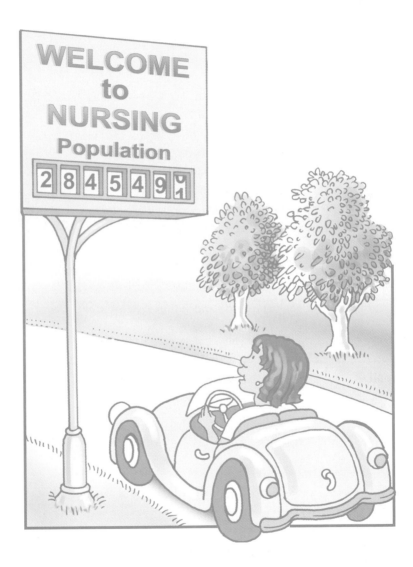

4

Destination: Registered Nurse

"Destiny is not a matter of chance, it is a matter of choice; it is not a thing to be waited for, it is a thing to be achieved."
—William Jennings Bryan

Welcome to nursing! It is the most exasperating career ever invented. It is also the most fulfilling. I can guarantee you intangible rewards that can rarely be matched by any other profession.

What I cannot guarantee are tangible rewards as rich as the intangible ones. Nursing is fraught with all the problems facing any job category that is manned predominantly by women.

Although I've written several books for nurses, the most popular piece I have written is the following poem. It is often read at pinning ceremonies and graduations.

BEING A NURSE MEANS . . .

You will never be bored.

You will often be frustrated.

You will be surrounded by challenges—so much to do and so little time.

You will carry immense responsibility with very little authority.

You will step into people's lives, and you will make a difference.

Some will bless you. Some will curse you.

You will see people at their worst—and at their best. You will never cease to be amazed at people's capacity for love, courage, and endurance.

You will see life begin and end.

You will experience resounding triumphs and devastating failures.

You will cry a lot.

You will laugh a lot.

You will know what it is to be human and to be humane.

What tangible rewards can you expect from nursing? The quickest way to assess your future earning potential is to look at the most current career opportunity guides published annually by nursing journal companies. Hospitals spend big bucks advertising in these guides, hoping to entice nurses to come work for them.

NURSING CAREER GUIDE DECODER KIT

As you investigate salaries, it may appear that there are some significant variations around the country. However, if you adjust those salaries in terms of cost of living, the differences effectively evaporate. For example, it costs twice as much to live half as well in New York City as it does in rural Georgia.

In the 2005 career guides, these were some of the perquisites hospitals were proud to offer:

"Day care on site"
"Relocation allowance up to $5000"
"37.5-hour work week"
"12 holidays per year"
"4 weeks of vacation"
"Half of all weekends off"
"Physical fitness center and pool"

"Tuition reimbursement for senior year"
"Up to $8000 for student loan forgiveness"
"NO SHIFT ROTATION"
"Uniform allowance"
"Loyalty bonus up to $500"
"Weekend bonus of 25%"
"Free parking"
"401(k) plan"
"Dental and vision insurance"
"Discounts on prescription drugs"
"Discount mortgages and home equity loans"
"Tax-sheltered annuities"
"Evening/night differentials" (ranging from less than
    $3000 to more than $12,000 per year)

Read between the lines. This is the good stuff. These hospitals are boasting. That means a lot of hospitals offer less vacation, fewer holidays, no tuition reimbursement, no uniform allowance, no bonuses for weekend work, no dental insurance, and little differential for working evenings or nights. It also means that many hospitals will require you to rotate shifts and to work more than half of the weekends.

You are not stupid. You know sick people need care around the clock, 7 days a week, 365 days a year, including weekends and holidays. However, you might not have considered what that would mean to *you* as a working nurse.

One hospital stated in its ad that "mandatory overtime" had been eliminated for nurses with 5 years of service. That means if you have been with the hospital for less than 5 years, you will be required to work overtime.

Today, hospitals are again offering incentives such as job sharing, flexible schedules, sick child care, spa memberships, free maid service, and even sign-on bonuses of cold, hard cash. In fact, the Air Force was advertising a $15,000 sign-on bonus.

A major change in incentives from the 2001 to the 2005 career guides was the emphasis on retaining nurses, not just recruiting them. Many had discontinued sign-on bonuses in favor of retention bonuses and other incentives for loyal nurses. Here are some examples:

"Comprehensive orientation with one-on-one preceptors"
"E-learning center with 24-hour access"
"Pristine state-of-the-art facilities"
"Great patient/nurse ratio"
"The flexibility you need to balance career and family time"
"Domestic partner insurance"
"Generous commitment incentives"
"Concierge services"
"On-site BSN and MSN programs"
"Fellowships and internships"
"Shared governance" (a management philosophy in which nurses are respected, included in decision making, and have control over their practice)

Nursing continues to provide better-than-average benefits for both its full-time and part-time workers in important areas such as health insurance, pension plans, sick days, and vacations than most other industries.

At the start of 2005, the average nurse, working full time in an acute care setting, was making about $55,000 a year. Starting salaries averaged between $34,000 and $48,000 a year, depending primarily on geographic area. Inexperienced nurses made from $19 to $24 per hour; experienced nurses, $28 to $59 per hour.

Compressed salary scales are less of a problem than they used to be. Not long ago, salary differences for inexperienced and experienced nurses varied as little as 10% to 15%. Today, there is a 30% to 50% difference.

What will nursing be like by the time you graduate? There's only one way to find out. Come along for the ride.

*"The price one pays for pursuing any profession or calling is
an intimate knowledge of its ugly side."*
—James Baldwin

*"A positive attitude will not solve all your problems, but it will
annoy enough people to make it worth the effort."*
—John Galsworthy

*"Life is a great big canvas, and you should throw all
the paint on it you can."*
—Danny Kay

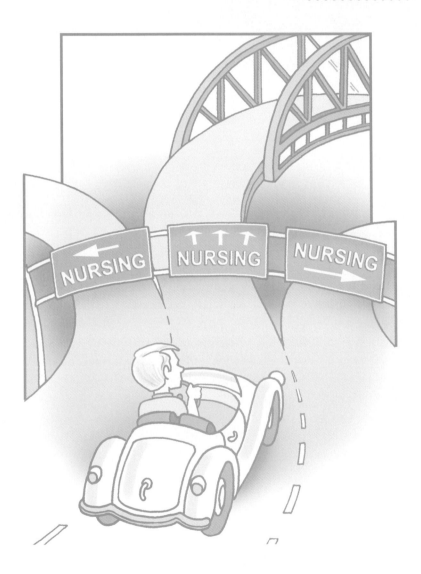

5

How Long Will This Trip Take?

"If you have built castles in the air, your work need not be lost; that is where they should be. Now put the foundations under them."
—Henry David Thoreau

"*A Genuine College Degree in 2 Weeks!*" This astonishing offer popped up in my e-mail.

The message went on to say: "Have you ever thought that the only thing stopping you from a great job and better pay was a few letters behind your name? Well now you can get them! Within 2 weeks! No study required! 100% verifiable! These are real, genuine degrees that include bachelor's, master's, and doctorate degrees\student records and transcripts are also available. This opportunity exists due to a legal loophole allowing some established colleges to award degrees at their discretion."

I was to call Claire and to call fast because she wouldn't be surprised to see this loophole closed very soon. Don't bother calling. I'd be surprised if Claire or her number were still working.

When you look for a nursing program, make sure you pick one that is "accredited" by the state and meets national nursing school standards. If you don't, you may lose a lot of time and money.

When you first learned that there are three different routes (associate degree, diploma, baccalaureate) to becoming a registered nurse, you may have decided to take the fastest, cheapest, most convenient route. After all, who in his or her right mind would spend twice as much time and money to end up with the same credential? A nurse is a nurse.

That is like saying a car is a car. Although the statement is essentially true, it is not the whole truth. For example, both a Volkswagen and a Mercedes are fine automobiles. Either will provide you with years of dependable transportation. The Mercedes, however, comes equipped with many options not available on economy cars.

If you are enrolled in an associate degree or diploma program, you will emerge driving an economy car. Good job opportunities will be available to you, but some career opportunities will be inaccessible unless you "trade up."

Many hospital salary scales reinforce the nurse-is-a-nurse theory. They may make little monetary distinction between nurses with and nurses without a bachelor's degree. However, those same hospitals often refuse to promote a staff nurse who lacks a BSN degree.

The debate over educational preparation for nurses has raged for decades and is hotly contested. It is the most divisive and potentially destructive issue facing nursing, which has made writing this chapter my most difficult challenge.

I have been a student in two of the three programs and a teacher in all of them. I would be the first to tell you that the length of the program is no guarantee of quality. Admirable programs and abominable programs exist at every level. It is all in the engineering.

After you finish your education, you will be required to complete a comprehensive set of exams to secure licensure as a registered nurse. To find how well your prospective nursing school is *engineered*, ask about its failure rates on state board examinations for the past 5 years. Until the last few years, a 5% failure rate meant "heads would roll"; the dean or director would be called on the carpet. Now the average failure rate is closer to 20%. Again, length of the program is not a factor. There are 2-year programs with a 0% failure rate and 4-year programs with a 37% failure rate. Make sure you go with a winner, or your trip could take much longer than expected. In fact, you might never arrive!

As I said, writing this chapter has been my most difficult challenge. Actually, when I hit on the Mercedes/Volkswagen analogy, I thought it was a stroke of genius, a clever way to discuss the difference and keep with the book's theme.

After the first edition of this book hit the market, however, an instructor called to say she thought comparing her program to a Volkswagen was insulting. Ouch! I didn't choose the Mercedes/Volkswagen analogy to insult anyone. I chose it for clarity and because they are the only cars I have ever owned.

I graduated from a diploma program in 1963 and bought a Volkswagen "Bug." That Bug served me well for thousands of miles and took me from the Midwest to the Northwest, where I earned my bachelor's degree and found my bachelor —Gary. We might still be driving Volkswagens today if things had not happened the way they did.

First, Gary's youngest brother was killed in an auto accident. Soon afterward, a fellow graduate student was horribly injured in a crash. We became concerned about safety and believed we needed a more substantial car, but we were not sure what kind.

Buying the Mercedes began as a joke. We would go to the Mercedes showroom after dark and press our noses against the glass. One night the showroom was open. A salesman invited us in to view a film, which revealed safety features for the car that were incredible.

We were "sold," but we were poor graduate students. Not to worry! The dealer had a demonstrator at a great price, and he would give us a larger amount in trade-in allowance on the Bug than I had paid for it 4 years earlier. The dealer would even finance it. However, we were encouraged to see about bank financing because the dealer's was one fourth of a percent higher.

The bankers laughed at us. We didn't have collateral, we had marginal incomes, and horror of horrors—what if I became pregnant?!? I assured them that was absolutely impossible because I was already pregnant. In fact, that was the reason we wanted a safer car.

Well, we bought that 1967 230S with dealer financing. Five months later, we brought our newborn son home from the hospital in it. Both our sons grew up and learned to drive in that car. We drove it for more than 20 years and 280,000 miles until it finally succumbed to rust and teenage abuse. Then it became an organ donor for a matching 230S.

With cars, as with most things in life, it has been my experience that over the long run, the best often costs less. As you select a school of nursing, look to the long run. Think options and safety features.

LOOKING BEYOND THE HORIZON

It is not a question of becoming a nurse. All three paths lead to nursing. The question is, What do you want to do after you become a nurse? What sort of job would you like to have 5 years after graduation? Ten years after graduation?

At this stage of your journey, projecting yourself that far into the future may be nigh unto impossible. Just becoming a nurse seems light years away. All you want to do is get that RN behind your name and get a job. Graduating from any nursing school will open the door to an excellent job. But some of you want a lot more than a job. Some of you already have very definite ideas of where you want to go once you enter nursing.

If you envision yourself as a public health nurse, clinical specialist, nurse practitioner, researcher, consultant, teacher, head nurse, or director of nursing services, you will need a baccalaureate degree. Yes, the price of a baccalaureate education is high, but the cost of not having one may be even higher. It all depends on where you want to go in nursing.

For most career-oriented nurses, a bachelor's degree is only the beginning. Many find that their chosen destination in nursing requires a trip to graduate school.

Our profession has lagged behind others in standardizing its educational requirements. Think about physical therapists, occupational therapists, dietitians, pharmacists, and social workers. All require the baccalaureate degree as minimal preparation, and many require a master's degree or above before full professional privileges are granted. For physicians, the baccalaureate degree is required before they are even eligible for entrance into their professional school. Nursing has some catching up to do.

What happens if you get an associate's degree in nursing or are a diploma graduate and somewhere down the road you decide you want more options? You take your "vehicle" back to the "factory" (college or university). Many colleges are purists. They will insist you cannot have a Mercedes chassis powered by a Volkswagen engine. They will offer to rebuild your vehicle completely if you can come up with enough money and approximately 3 more years of your life. Other colleges act more like body shops. They will be happy to customize your vehicle for less time and money.

Few students receive adequate counseling before they choose a school of nursing. They often learn about the advantages and disadvantages of their particular program in their last semester. Think carefully about the options you want and what you can "afford," not just in terms of dollars but also in terms of time and distance.

Actually, most of your instructors and many of the nurses you will come to admire are driving some of the most incredible contraptions you can imagine. Check their backgrounds and credentials. You will see that your basic preparation will not determine how far you can go in nursing, but it will affect the amount of time it takes to get there.

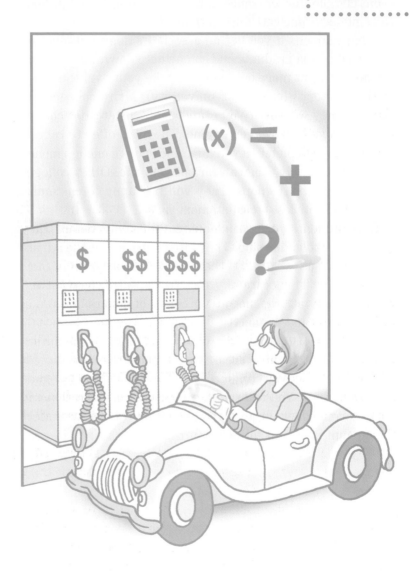

6

How Much Will This Trip Cost?

"Look at me: I worked my way up from nothing to a state of extreme poverty."
—Groucho Marx, *Monkey Business*

*B*efore starting any trip, it is wise to estimate the costs. Otherwise, you may end up stranded and not only penniless, but deep in debt.

There are more than 1500 nursing programs in the United States. The cost can range from under $3000 a year at a community college to more than $40,000 a year at a private college. These costs reflect tuition only. They do not include room and board and such miscellaneous costs as books, uniforms, special equipment, travel, and laboratory fees. The cost of books, for example, averages more than $600 per year. (Your first-year book bill may be significantly higher because many of the books required in the freshman year are used throughout the entire program.)

When estimating costs, don't forget to include such incidentals as transportation to and from the clinical area, babysitters, and eating on the run.

One major cost often overlooked is that of deferred income—money you would have made if you had worked instead of going to school. If you allow $20,000 per year (a salary of $10 per hour), you can quickly see that the cost of *not working* will be $40,000 or $60,000 or $80,000, depending on whether you are enrolled in an associate degree, diploma, or baccalaureate program.

How much will *your* trip to nursing cost? Sit down with

your classmates and discuss all the potential costs, including deferred income. Work through the following exercise. The total figure will be quite a jolt.

Cost estimates of spending _____ years at _____
school of nursing

Tuition	_____
Room and board	_____
Books	_____
Uniform/special equipment	_____
Laboratory fees	_____
Transportation	_____
Deferred income	_____
Other:	
_____	_____
_____	_____
_____	_____
TOTAL	_____

Of course, there are ways to defray costs. You may be eligible for a scholarship, grant, or loan. Scholarships are usually given for academic achievement, whereas grants are based strictly on financial need. Student loans tend to carry very low interest charges, and repayment is not required until after graduation. Unlike loans, scholarships and grants do not have to be repaid.

MEGABUCKS IN MOTION

To find money to help finance your education, start with Johnson & Johnson's website *http://www.discovernursing. com.* I grew up in Iowa so I thought it would be fun to see what nursing programs are available there. The website found 34 programs for me. It gave me basic statistics about each one, listed their websites, and had a hot button to "Find scholarships to match this program."

Don't be shy. Ask local hospitals, auxiliaries, nursing associations, service clubs, and fraternal orders about their scholarship programs. Check the public library. Even if you are 40 years old, call your local high school counselor for advice. Don't forget the armed forces. They have some excellent scholarship and financial aid benefits. Valuable information may also be obtained by contacting the National League for Nursing, the American Nurses Association (ANA), your state chapter of the ANA, the National Student Nurses' Association, and the Canadian Nurses Association. (Addresses can be found in Appendixes B, C, and D.)

Monies are available from both the public and the private sectors. Because eligibility requirements and dollar amounts change annually, your best source of current information will be the financial aid office at your nursing school. You may also be eligible for a work-study program. Remember, just because you didn't start with a scholarship, grant, or loan doesn't mean you can't get one. Some monies become available only after you complete lower-division courses. Appendix B contains addresses you need to find out more about undergraduate financial aid and student loan programs.

Nursing students have taken out second mortgages, borrowed against insurance policies, and sold their boats, cars, and motorcycles to finance their education. A middle-aged student obtained a loan from her mother because "Mom always wanted me to become a nurse and she thought it was better late than never!" Another student said she was in school on "found" money. Once she decided to go to school, she found there were a lot of things she could do without.

How would you like to go to nursing school for free? Not only that, how would you like to be guaranteed a job with a great starting salary and fringe benefits? When a hospital in Pennsylvania made that offer, 48 students immediately signed up for the program. Many hospitals will pay off student loans or reimburse tuition expenses if you will agree to work there for a year or two.

At a national nursing convention, I had a great conversation with a fortysomething nurse. The next day she brought her twentysomething daughter, also a nurse, to meet me.

I congratulated her on recruiting her daughter into our profession. "Oh, no," they said in unison. The mother hadn't recruited the daughter. The *daughter* had recruited the mother. Thinking her mom would be a great nurse, she offered to pay mom's tuition. And, if mom made a "B" average, she didn't have to pay her daughter back!

Most of you are comparison shoppers. You try to get top value for each dollar spent. You watch for sales, clip coupons, and drive miles out of the way to save a few bucks.

When it comes to educational dollars, however, some students behave in a most irrational manner. They would never dream of going to the store and asking the clerk, "What's the least I can get for 20 bucks?" Yet they plunk their tuition money down and then ask the instructor, "What's the least I can get for this and still graduate?" They concentrate on the minimum requirements instead of reaching for the maximum.

Regardless of what financial aid you manage to muster, this educational experience is still going to cost you thousands and thousands of dollars. So approach education in a businesslike manner. You have "contracted" with the school for certain services. Make sure it delivers. You have "hired" these instructors. Be sure to get what you have paid for by learning and experiencing everything you can.

Be a smart consumer. Get your money's worth.

The cost of a nursing education cannot be measured in dollars alone. Another price will be paid in blood, sweat, and tears.

NOW THEY KNOW

I asked students attending a National Student Nurses' Association convention to share one thing they wish they had known before deciding to major in nursing. Here are some of their answers:

"ONE THING I WISH I HAD KNOWN *BEFORE* I CHOSE TO MAJOR IN NURSING IS

... how difficult it was going to be!"
... how much reading there is."
... how much paperwork there is to do!"

... that so much outside work was required."

... that even though I was an honor student in high school, college is totally different."

... how much actual work it requires! (Or maybe I'm glad I didn't know. I might not have finished.)"

... that I would need to keep white underwear in stock for the rest of my life."

... how to prepare for the shock and trauma of the nursing class/clinical schedule."

... that fraternities may have 'Hell Week' but nursing has 'Hell Years.'"

... about nursing school side effects—sexual dysfunction, sleeplessness, night terrors, restlessness. Then again, maybe I'm better having not known!"

... the astonishing amount of knowledge you must gain in 4 years."

... what nursing really is."

... what nurses really do."

... more about the three different ways to become an R.N."

... all about the entry into practice issue! I certainly would have appreciated the honesty."

... the expense!"

... that you are no longer an individual until you graduate— you belong to the nursing program, physically and spiritually. On graduation you develop wings and fly."

... the number of clinical options available."

... how much time I would be investing (I'm married) and how much discipline I would need (and how much weight I was going to gain!)."

... how important computers and technology are."

... that at 43 years of age I would feel so completely awkward and useless. But by the beginning of the next year, I felt empowered and smart!"

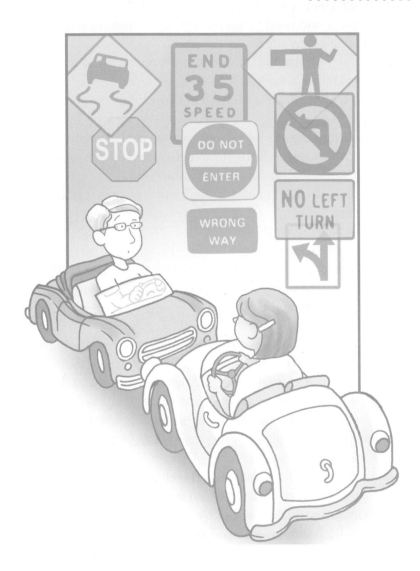

7

Rules of the Road

"Each is given a bag of tools,
A shapeless mass,
A book of rules;
And each must make,
Ere life is flown,
A stumbling-block
Or a stepping-stone."
—R. L. Sharpe, "Stumbling-Block or Stepping-Stone"

All schools of nursing are similar, but no two are identical. Each has designed its own highly customized track on which you will learn how to be a nurse.

Upon your admission, the school effectively issues you a learner's permit. If you fail to follow the rules of its road, your permit may be canceled. Therefore knowing the rules and regulations is imperative.

So ... READ THE RULES. Take a deep breath and read them again. Ignorance can cost you big bucks and add months to your program. Don't be caught saying, "I didn't know ... I had to have organic chemistry first ... my incomplete would automatically convert to an F... Abnormal Psychology was only offered winter quarter ... three clinical absences meant I had to repeat the course ... advanced registration began last week ... fees were due Monday."

Check the college catalog, the student handbook, special orientation packets, and all first-day-of-class handouts. Don't just read them; study them. Underline vital information and make notes in the margins. Highlight those things that apply to you immediately or in the near future. If you have questions, get clarification. Don't rely on the grapevine for the latest word on course requirements. Go directly to the source. Talk with the instructor involved.

These policies were not written by God, but they might as well have been. They do not reflect spur-of-the-moment decisions. They are decisions that have evolved over many years. Countless deans, directors, faculty members, students, advisory boards, and ad hoc committees have devised and revised the rules and regulations governing your school of nursing.

If the rules and regulations begin to get you down, remember that what appears to be a roadblock may actually be a guardrail placed there to keep you from plunging off a cliff.

RULES AND REASONS

Schools of nursing represent a huge investment in manpower and machinery. Their programs are among the most expensive to run. They are insured to the hilt and are accountable to more governmental and professional agencies than you can imagine. They will supply you with teachers, classrooms, laboratories, disposable equipment, and not-so-disposable patients. The schools shoulder an enormous responsibility. In return, you must grant them a few eccentricities.

For example, most schools have written codes for dress and behavior. This really irks some students. They consider it an infringement on their personal rights. It is nothing personal. It is strictly professional. This may be the first time your personal freedoms collide with professional responsibilities, but it won't be the last.

Before bursting into a chorus of "I've Gotta Be Me," consider the advantages of being "me" on your own time. You can avoid all sorts of headaches and hassles if you simply agree to bathe regularly, use deodorant, wear shoes, spit out your chewing gum, or give up showing off your latest body piercing.

On the school's time, be a polished professional. On your own time, cut loose, relax, and enjoy. At first you may feel absolutely schizophrenic. Gradually, the "real" you and the "professional" you will meld and mature into a "new" you.

If you want to stay in school, CONFORM. Sure, you can fight the system. But face it, you don't have the time, energy, or cunning it takes to win. You'll just end up spinning your wheels while other students drive off with diplomas.

Instead of fighting the system, use it. When conflicts arise, take your concerns, suggestions, and grievances to the student-faculty committee responsible for such matters. Then hurry back to the business of learning. After all, your job is not to revamp this school of nursing. Your job is to graduate.

There is no such thing as a perfect school of nursing, an optimum curriculum, or an ideal textbook. But we are working on it. That is why you will find curricula constantly under construction, courses being remodeled, textbooks being switched midyear, and learning experiences that seem to appear and disappear without warning. Be sure to see your advisor regularly to be aware of any upcoming changes as well as to keep tabs on your progress.

One student inquired about a computer course labeled 108X. Although the description sounded like just what she needed, she noticed that no other course in that column had an "X rating." She was told it denoted an experimental course that was "not quite approved." She wisely chose another course that was fully approved.

When you are handed an armload of paper listing miles of rules and regulations, it is hard to believe that all of this has been compiled to make student life less complicated. On careful examination, however, you'll find that these papers do more than outline your obligations: they safeguard your opportunities. Following the instructions makes your graduation not only a possibility but a distinct probability.

Yes, there are exceptions to every rule. But are you really that exceptional?

"This is the grave of Mike O'Day
Who died maintaining his right of way.
His right was clear, his will was strong,
But he's just as dead as if he'd been wrong."
—Epitaph

8

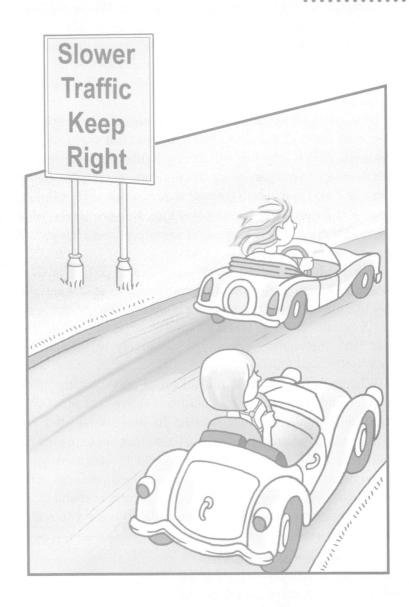

Slower Traffic Keep Right

"Nothing is more terrible than ignorance in action."
—Johann Wolfgang von Goethe

*I*f you are just starting out on your first lap around the track, listen to some student-to-student tips for success. Students attending a National Student Nurses' Association convention were asked to share one "survival" tip they would like to pass on to beginning students.

Their suggestions can be divided into four categories: (1) take care of yourself; (2) take care of each other; (3) take one day at a time; and (4) take care of business.

TAKE CARE OF YOURSELF

"Set time aside each day for yourself or your family."
"Don't spend all of your time studying."
"Make sure to take care of yourself. Don't put nursing school ahead of your own health."
"Make sure you look your best every day. The better you look, the better others will treat you."
"Eat breakfast."
"The best advice in the world is don't take advice from anyone. You are a unique individual and your experience in nursing school will be unique as well."
"Be involved in more activities on campus than just nursing school. It helps keep your sanity."
"As our mothers always told us, you are who you hang with! Stay with people who make you feel good about

yourself—no negativity. Negativity drains the soul and the mind. Any obstacle can be overcome with an open mind and a positive attitude."

"Take dance breaks while studying. It will keep you energized and in a good mood."

"Take a fun elective."

"Study hard, but play hard too. Make time for friends. Take walks, work out, dance, swim, play tennis—it will keep you sane."

"Science and math can be learned. Caring can't. Don't let chemistry and pharmacology intimidate you and keep you from becoming a nurse!"

"Have friends outside of the nursing department—clubs, athletics, churches. Friends who are not in nursing help you get your mind off things. They are wonderful!"

"No matter how much advice you get, it won't matter unless you take it, apply it, live with it, and most important, USE IT!"

TAKE CARE OF EACH OTHER

"Build a support system with your fellow students."

"Work together as a class. Don't let the competitive spirit get in the way."

"Get involved early with NSNA (National Student Nurses' Association). Networking is important."

"Join a study group. I couldn't have made it without mine."

"The steps to good nursing: RAID without the bugs! R = Read material carefully. A = Apply what was learned. I = Instruct fellow classmates who do not understand. D = Demonstrate your learning during clinical practice."

"I have adult attention deficit disorder. What works for me is a group of four to five students where everyone reads a section of the material and that person explains the material to the group. Or compare the same information in different books and discuss it in the group until everyone understands."

"Study with friends. Try studying for 50 minutes and
   playing or talking for 10 minutes. Repeat. It's not much
   of a social life, but it's better than nothing."
"Get involved with other students. They can help you, and
   you can help them."

TAKE ONE DAY AT A TIME

"Take it one day, one test, one patient at a time, and don't
   get discouraged."
"Don't take introductory classes too seriously. They are
   meant to weed out students. Hang in there until clinical.
   You'll love it!"
"When you first enter school, write down all your reasons
   for going into nursing. Keep the list where you can see it
   every day. It will keep you from giving up when you hit
   a rough patch."
"Don't worry when you feel like you are behind: you are!
   But so is everyone else. Don't give up!"
"Live one day at a time. Once something is done, don't
   worry about it. Just keep doing your best at each task."
"Make the best of any situation by adjusting your attitude."
"Please yourself—be happy meeting your own
   personal/professional/academic goals."
"I was the mother of five young children when I went to
   nursing school. If I can do it, anyone can!"
"Looking at the overall picture can be pretty scary. Just
   concentrate on one assignment at a time."

TAKE CARE OF BUSINESS

"MAKE NURSING SCHOOL YOUR FIRST PRIORITY."
"Take classes seriously. Start out studying hard."
"Maintain good study habits."
"Keep up with the reading from day one."
"Do the reading as you go along. Don't wait!"
"Take the extra time needed to do extra readings."
"Read, read, read. Study, study, study. Read some more.
   Study some more. Don't stop!"

KEEP UP WITH WORK RATHER THAN TRYING TO CATCH UP

"Start a good home library to use for care plans."

"Keep your notes current."

"Review notes daily."

"Organize your time. Conserve your energy."

"No significant others—unless they are science majors!"

"Use Sunday night to plan your entire week."

"Create your own flash cards."

"Be prepared for three times more work than you ever imagined."

"Type your class notes. It will help you remember."

"Take a course in stress management."

"Don't take yourself seriously. Take your commitments seriously."

"Let everyone else worry about the politics and all the other stuff YOU CAN'T CONTROL! Stay focused on your studies and what YOU CAN CONTROL!"

"In the clinical area, volunteer to help with anything— be a 'gopher' for your nurse."

"Build up your GPA before you start taking all nursing courses."

"Learn to be happy with Cs and thrilled with Bs (especially if you were a straight-A student in high school)."

"Keep all your ducks in a row so you don't quack up!"

"Get a tutor if necessary."

"Rip out the section of the book you are currently reading, put it in a plastic folder, and put the appropriate class notes with it. It will save your back and you can read it in the bathroom!"

"Do not take too many sciences in one semester."

"Make sure you're financially stable enough to work minimal hours while in school."

"Have enough food in your freezer for a year!"

"Realize that it is impossible to work full time and be a good student. If you want to survive nursing, don't try to work full time."

"Get to know your instructors."

"Make sure your teachers know you—your name, your
    face—you. Not your number. It makes all the
    difference."

"Do what the teacher tells you to do. Don't argue; just do it!
    It will decrease your stress and your teacher's stress
    too."

"Buy a book on nursing math and bone up ahead of time."

"Don't just memorize material. Learn how to apply it."

"Ninety percent of what you learn you teach yourself.
    Practice! Practice! Practice! Spend as much time as you
    can in the lab practicing those procedures. Role-playing
    works."

"When your patient tells you something like, '*This is the
    best place to start an IV,*' *LISTEN!*'"

"Keep your sense of humor!"

"Learn how to live without sleep."

"Don't forget to breathe."

Ready? Set? Go! Take the on ramp and don't look back.
Just go slowly and stay in the right lane.

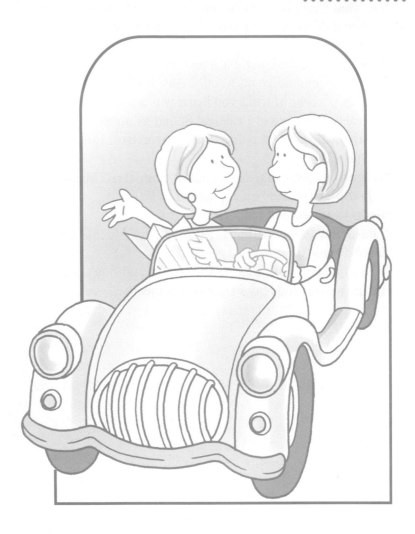

9

Driving Instructors

"We judge ourselves by what we feel capable of doing, while others judge us by what we have already done."
—Henry Wadsworth Longfellow

Meet your driving instructors. These are the experts you've hired to take you over the course. Get to know them. Remember that they are people first, nurses second, and teachers third.

Get to know them as people. They are human. They are not infallible, omniscient, or omnipotent. They have their likes and dislikes, their dreams and fears, their good days and bad days, their strengths and weaknesses. They have diverse cultural, familial, religious, and geographic backgrounds. Each has a different philosophy of life.

Get to know them as nurses. Find out what attracted them to nursing in the first place, where they were educated, what their clinical specialties are, where they have worked, which professional organizations they belong to, what articles or books they have written, and what their goals are. Each has a different philosophy of nursing.

Get to know them as teachers. Find out how long they have been teaching, where else they have taught, what their favorite subject matter is, and in which clinical areas they enjoy guiding students. Some instructors see themselves as scholars and researchers. Others see themselves as catalysts, facilitators, role models, or even recruiters for the nursing profession. Each has a different philosophy of teaching.

Your goal is not to "psych out" the instructors so you can get by with learning as little as possible. Your goal is to "psych out" the instructors so you can learn as much as possible.

CHOICE OF INSTRUCTORS

By identifying instructors compatible with your needs, goals, philosophy, and style, you can make learning much easier. For example, if you prefer freedom to examine, experience, and discover information for yourself, you will suffocate under an instructor who delivers formal lectures and insists that everyone stay together in lock-step fashion. On the other hand, if you are a student who prefers a lot of structure and no surprises, you might excel under such an instructor.

Avoid instructors with whom you are dreadfully mismatched in terms of style, philosophy, or temperament. If you find yourself in such a situation, decide whether you can successfully adapt or should seek an immediate transfer. Avoid any instructor who boasts of being a harsh grader. Always remember that your number one goal is to graduate.

Keep your eyes open for instructors who are masters of their craft, intellectually stimulating, and accessible in times of trouble. Instructors are prone to clone, so stick close to those you would like to resemble when you grow up (professionally speaking).

"A teacher affects eternity; he can never tell where his influence stops."
—Henry Adams, *The Education of Henry Adams*

Most instructors hold advanced degrees and, in the course of obtaining those degrees, have become highly specialized. That is why teaching teams are so common in schools of nursing. A team of instructors picks you up at point X and delivers you to point Y, where another team of specialists takes over. It's rather like a cross between a road rally and a relay race.

ONE FOR THE ROAD

Whenever you encounter a new set of instructors, always assume the best. "These instructors are here to help me.

They sincerely want me to succeed. They will do everything they can on my behalf." Even in the face of evidence to the contrary, assume the best.

Positive attitudes are contagious. Instructors enjoy working with students who are optimistic, courteous, cooperative, self-disciplined, responsible, respectful, and proud of the work they are doing. The more of these attributes you have, the more successful you will be.

Negative attitudes are equally contagious. If you are pessimistic, uncooperative, hesitant, or uninterested, your nonverbal behavior will give away your inner thoughts. The instructors will have an uneasy feeling about you. They will begin to question your ability, and your chances of failure will be greater.

Who lives longer: pessimists or optimists? In the 1960s the Mayo Clinic routinely gave the Minnesota Multiphasic Personality Inventory (MMPI) test to its patients. One element of the MMPI was an optimism-pessimism scale. It seems that 15% of the test takers were optimists, 15% were pessimists, and the other 70% were somewhere in the middle.

Thirty years later someone must have been rummaging around in the files and thought it would be interesting to see if there were any correlation between optimism, pessimism, and longevity. I guess we'll never know. The researcher tried to talk with the pessimists, but they were dead.

Your relationship with your nursing instructors will mirror your relationships with authority figures in general. Think about how you relate to parents, clergy, employers, police officers, and other authorities. Do you see them as friends or foes? Are you usually agreeable or argumentative? Suspicious or trusting?

There are only two totally unreasonable nursing instructors in the entire country. Invariably, one will be employed by your school of nursing. If you think you are dealing with more than one totally unreasonable instructor, you have a problem. You are either in the wrong school, the wrong profession, or both.

TEACHER/LEARNER/STUDENT/NURSE

You may be surprised to learn that many of your nursing instructors are students themselves. Many are working on advanced degrees. They have to write term papers and take final exams. They have to worry about their own GPAs as well as yours.

Just as the nursing profession is moving toward standardizing its educational requirements to be on a par with other professions, nursing education is moving toward requiring the same credentials held by college professors in other departments.

Only a few years ago in many schools of nursing, a bachelor's degree was considered adequate preparation for many teaching positions. Today, teaching opportunities for nurses with bachelor's degrees are few and fleeting. Occasionally, these nurses are hired to help teach in the clinical setting on a temporary basis. For most faculty members, a master's degree is required, and doctoral preparation is preferred. At many colleges and universities, master's-prepared nurses are being phased out unless they are actively working toward a doctorate.

Having to be teacher and graduate student simultaneously is only one pressure felt by nursing faculty. In addition to their teaching duties, nursing faculty are also expected to engage in research, to publish widely, to be politically active, to perform community service, and to maintain competence in their clinical areas. Try adding marriage, children, or both to all of this and you have a better understanding of why faculty members are not always as accessible or patient as you would like them to be.

ROLES ROYCE

On the rocky road through nursing, your instructors will play many roles. As TOUR GUIDES they will plan the itinerary, provide maps, and staff the information booth. They will lead you through unfamiliar territory, introducing you to local customs, acting as interpreters, and making sure you don't offend the natives. Because they know what's coming around each bend, they will make sure you don't miss anything. By sharing stories and anecdotes, they weave together the past, present, and future of nursing.

As CONSTRUCTION WORKERS they pave the way so you can pass quickly and safely. They flag you around potholes and other possible pitfalls. They fill in gaps, build bridges, and lay good foundations. They know that before new structures can be built, old ones must sometimes be demolished. They help you bulldoze old attitudes, habits, prejudices, and other misinformation.

As HIGHWAY PATROL OFFICERS they police the road for your patients' protection. They not only handle emergencies and accidents, they also help prevent them by enforcing rules and regulations. They make sure everyone is going in the right direction at the right speed. If you break the rules, they may let you off with a warning, or they may issue a formal citation that lands you in front of the judge.

As TRAFFIC COURT JUDGES they listen to individual cases and hear appeals. They may place you on probation, fine you, or suspend your license to learn. Not all of an instructor's tasks are pleasant, but all are necessary.

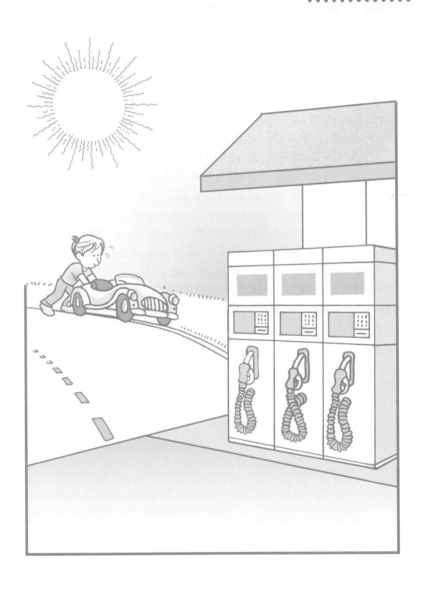

10

More Miles per Gallon

"Genius is one percent inspiration and ninety-nine percent perspiration."
—Thomas Edison

*T*hink of the hours in your week as gallons of gas in your tank. Every student has precisely the same amount, yet some get much farther on their weekly tank of gas than others.

If you want to get more miles per gallon, there are two things you must do. You must learn to be more EFFICIENT and more EFFECTIVE. Being more efficient means learning to do things right. Being more effective means learning to do the right things.

When it comes to efficiency, you can get more mileage by improving your reading and writing skills than any other way. Do whatever is necessary to increase your proficiency (see "Reading and Remembering" in Chapter 13). These skills will not only bring success to you as a student, they will also give you the leading edge as a professional in years to come.

Front-running students know how to conserve fuel. They know that the difference between studying for short periods and studying for long periods is like the difference between city and highway driving. They know they will accomplish more, faster, and with less wear and tear on their machinery if they take studying up to cruising speed and hold it there for an hour, or two, or three.

But no matter how efficient you become, you still will not get where you want to go if you drive off in the wrong direction. That is where effectiveness comes into play. You not only need to read well, you need to read right—the right books, the right chapters, the right journals. You may be a faster writer and technically flawless yet write wrong—the wrong topics, the wrong themes, the wrong conclusions.

How do you know what's right and what's wrong? Ask your instructor. Listen carefully.

IMPROVING YOUR FUEL EFFICIENCY

Another way students manage to get more miles to the gallon is by driving economy models. They operate under a principle described by an ancient Italian economist named Pareto. His 80/20 principle, loosely translated, says that 80% of the value or satisfaction will come from 20% of the tasks or activities.

So if you have ten things to do today, two of them will account for 80% of the day's success. Leading students are able to look at their "to do" lists and zero in on the two or three activities that have the highest payoff potential. They tackle those first. If there is time left, they take care of some of the remaining items.

Floundering students make no distinction regarding the payoff value of items on their "to do" lists. They begin anywhere, usually with the easiest items. By the end of the day, they have accomplished eight of the ten items on their list. Unfortunately, they did the eight that gave them only a 20% return on their time.

Using this proportional approach when setting priorities has some very practical applications. For example, if your instructor is a specialist in the subject matter, 80% of the test will come from lecture and only 20% will come from the readings. However, if the instructor is a specialist in cardiac care but has to pinch-hit in a psychiatric nursing course, 80% of the test will come from the readings and only 20% will come from lecture.

Once you become aware of the 80/20 principle, you will begin to see all sorts of other applications. You will notice that 80% of your homework comes from 20% of your teachers, that 80% of all prescriptions involve only 20% of the drugs, and that 80% of what you need to know is contained in 20% of your textbook. Ah … if only you knew which 20%!

Superstudents have developed the ability to pick out the 20% of the reading that gives them 80% of what they need to know. They don't try to master everything in the textbook. They concentrate on that small percentage that allows them to sail through exams and to perform competently in the clinical area. If you need help developing this ability, see Chapter 13, "Drive-Up Teller."

Here are some other tips to help you get more miles per gallon.

TIME MANAGEMENT FROM A TO Z FOR NURSING STUDENTS

ATTENDANCE. Every hour you spend in class will save you 3 hours of study time. If you are going to cut corners somewhere, go to class and skimp on study time. Attend every class.

BUDGETING. Most students claim they just don't have enough time. Yet every student has all the time there is: 168 hours per week, no more and no less. Therefore managing your time becomes even more important than managing your money because once time is spent, you can't earn more.

To make sure you use each day to the maximum, buy a pocket-sized daily planner or an electronic personal digital assistant (PDA) and keep it with you. If necessary, buy a jumbo calendar to keep track of major events. Scope the whole term, marking out such milestones as exams, term papers, and research projects. Block out all clinical times. Don't forget to allow time for preclinical work such as reading charts, making care plans, and interviewing patients.

Approach being a student as you would a job. Plan to be at it 40 hours a week. Small business owners will tell you they average closer to 60 hours a week, and you qualify as a small business.

Don't make the mistake of thinking that because you have only one class on Tuesday and no class on Thursday, those are your "days off." Actually, those are the days when you can really get down to business. Although it is important to use every fragment of time, it is even more important to schedule large blocks of uninterrupted study time lasting 2 or 3 hours.

CONCENTRATION. One key to success is undivided attention. Eliminate all distractions. Clear your work area and your mind of all clutter. Keep on the desk only what you need for a particular assignment. If your mind wanders, order it back to the task at hand. Superstudents not only do first things first, they do only one thing at a time.

DIRTY JOBS. Look at your "to do" list and circle the task you dread doing most. Tackle that one first. When it is finished, you will feel exhilarated.

If you postpone doing a boring, tough, or unpleasant task, it will nag you all day. Your ability to concentrate will be nil. As the day wears on, you will begin to think about putting it off until tomorrow. That way the task will ruin two days instead of one. So take the plunge and do the dirty job first.

EQUIPMENT. Have a ready supply of pens, pencils, paper, note cards, computer disks, and printer ribbons or cartridges on hand. There is nothing more inconvenient than having to make a mad dash to an all-night convenience store.

Invest in the latest edition of each required textbook. Should you buy a used book? Buying a pre-owned book is like buying a used car. If the previous owner was a straight-A student, the yellow highlights and scribbles in the margins may be a godsend. Unfortunately, most straight-

A students keep their books. The market is flooded with C-minus students' books. If your eye is easily distracted by another student's notes or highlighting, buy a new book.

To avoid frequent trips to the library for minor tidbits of information, build your own mini-reference library. Besides a standard dictionary and thesaurus, include a medical/nursing dictionary, drug handbook, Merck Medical Manual, and _____ . (Ask your instructors for suggestions to fill in the blank.)

FILING SYSTEM. With the "it-must-be-here-somewhere" filing system, you will not only lose time, you will lose your temper. Browse at the local bookstore for a filing system that meets your needs. If you can't afford what's in the store, go behind the store and get a sturdy cardboard box from the trash. Keep everything together. Put all papers pertaining to a certain class in one folder, and keep all folders for the current term in one box.

Once the term is over, take all those folders and move them to an under-the-bed storage box. That way the stuff will be out of sight but easily accessible. Then when your classroom studies are focused on the renal system, but you find yourself caring for a pregnant schizophrenic with a broken leg, you can quickly find your notes from last term or even last year.

GOALS. Goals may be as simple as reading two chapters before bedtime or as complex as becoming a *nurse-midwife* in Borneo. Some take 10 minutes to accomplish; others take 10 years.

Being goal-oriented helps you focus your time and energy for maximum effect. It enables you to weed out irrelevant people and activities. Dozens of daily decisions become automatic.

If you find yourself wishing you could get a better grade in anatomy and physiology, or get into the clinical rotation at Children's Hospital next spring, or get more help with the housework, stop wishing and convert those wishes into goals. Sit down and work through the following:

1. List the steps you need to take to achieve the goal.
2. Decide which steps you are able to take to achieve the goal.
3. Decide which steps you are willing to take to achieve the goal.
4. Identify people who can help you achieve the goal.
5. Consider how you might let yourself or others sabotage your good intentions.

If you take the time to write down a goal and your plan for achieving it, you won't need a fairy godmother to make your dreams come true.

HANGING IN THERE. When the going gets tough, hang in there. As the difficulty of any task increases, so does the attractiveness of any distraction. As you squirm in your chair, doing your laundry suddenly seems vital. Ignore the laundry. Knuckle down and work through the problem at hand. If you abandon a task when you feel you are losing, you'll find it much harder to return to it. Active avoidance coupled with passive procrastination will cost you lots of time. Instead, stop work at a point where you feel you are winning. Then you will be willing, even eager, to return to the task later.

INVESTMENTS. Think of class attendance, library time, and study sessions as "deposits." Even brief moments, like small change, can add up to something big. One student tucked chemical formulas into her ski boot and memorized them on the chairlift.

Learn to prioritize. Invest time in high-payoff activities. Required classes take priority over electives. Nursing classes take priority over any other class. Studying for an exam that makes up 50% of your grade takes precedence over studying for an exam that only makes up 10% of a grade. And so on.

JOTTING IT DOWN. Make lists and use them. It's the best way to stay organized and avoid wasted motion. Lists help you consolidate errands so that you make two trips instead of 20. Lists help you arrive prepared and ready for action.

Efficiency experts suggest you make a list each evening for the following day. List the six most critical things that have to be done. Rank them in order of importance. The next day, begin with number one and work it through before going on to anything else. Continue down the list. Your productivity will skyrocket.

KNOCKING OFF. When you reach the point of diminishing returns, discontinue an activity. Settle for an A—don't knock your brains out striving for an A-plus. No one wastes more time than a perfectionist.

Remember Parkinson's Law: "Work expands to fill the amount of time available to do it." Set reasonable deadlines and stick to them. Then move on to the next task.

LIBRARIAN. No one on campus can help you save as much time as the librarian. Just ask.

MAJORING IN MINOR ACTIVITIES. Busywork gives many students a false sense of accomplishment. Each night they fall into bed exhausted, insisting they are working as hard as they can. They're right. They're just not working as smart as they can.

Learn to recognize busywork for what it is. Don't take pride in your efforts. Take pride only in results.

"NO." The greatest timesaving device ever invented.

OTHER PEOPLE'S TIME. Time-wise students know how to divide chores and delegate everything they possibly can. They are also aware of some important considerations when relying on other people's time.

For example, if you are hiring someone to type your term paper, get the material to the typist well in advance of the due date. One campus typist, tired of last-minute hysterics, posted this notice on her wall: "A LACK OF PLANNING ON YOUR PART DOES NOT CONSTITUTE AN EMERGENCY ON MINE." If you are relying on other people's time, plan far ahead.

PRIME TIME. Every person has 2 or 3 hours a day when he or she is in top form. Most of us have our prime time in the morning.

Find your prime time and protect it. Invest it in high-priority items that demand concentration, creativity, and judgment. Use your less-than-prime time for legwork.

QUESTIONS. Several times each day, ask yourself questions such as the following:

- Is this the best use of my time right now?
- Is this activity helping me achieve one of my goals?
- Is this worth the amount of time it will take?
- Is this still worth doing?
- If I didn't do this, what would happen?

REGRETS. Don't squander time mourning what might have been. Don't waste time wallowing in guilt or self-pity. When you begin to say, "If only _____ ," quickly change the statement to "Next time _____." Then get on with the business at hand.

SAVING TIME. Impossible! It is also impossible to find time or make time. You can only put the time you have to better use.

TOMORROW. It never comes. Do it TODAY.

URGENCY! Urgent things are not always important. Important things are not always urgent. Tending to the important and ignoring the pseudoimportant things that clamor for attention are what separate good students from great students.

VACILLATING. Indecision robs students of enough time to be classified as grand larceny. Be decisive. Establish your own operating policies. If you give yourself a deadline, stick to it. If you decide your regular study period will be from 2:00 to 4:00 PM, Monday through Friday, don't violate that policy. Studying anything is better than studying nothing.

WASTEBASKET. Use it!

XEROXING. For dimes and quarters you can cut your library time to the bone. Use your less-than-prime time to round up all appropriate books and journals. Scan 2 minutes for articles, 3 minutes for books. Photocopy anything that appears pertinent. Use your prime time to study, memorize, integrate, synthesize, and use the information.

Keep copies of all your written papers and major assignments. If you prepared your assignment on a computer, be sure to save your work to the hard drive and a floppy disk or CD. It's a dirt-cheap insurance policy against loss.

YAKETY YAK. Don't let the telephone or a drop-in visitor ruin your study time. Tell callers, "I can't talk right now. I'll call you back at 9 o'clock." If you can't do that, unplug the phone or go where there are no phones.

Close your door. If someone pops in and asks, "Have you got a minute?" say "No, but I'll have a minute at 9 o'clock." Offer to meet in his or her room or in the coffee shop. That way you can control the length of the visit.

ZZZZS. Schedule rest-and-relaxation periods. Get the sleep you need so you will be alert enough to put all these time management suggestions to good use.

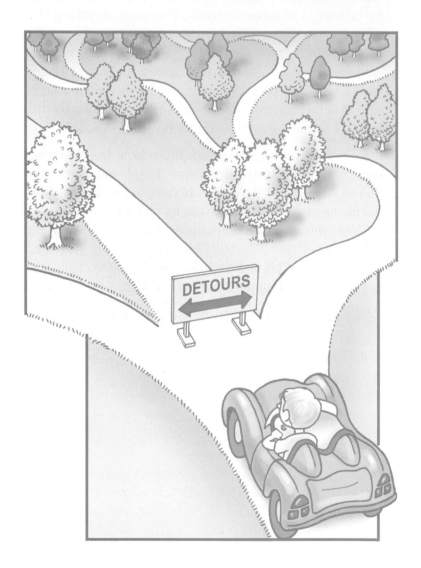

Detours

"Lost time is never found again."
—Benjamin Franklin, *Poor Richard's Almanac*

Clutching your "TO DO" list, you start off with the best intentions. Today you are really going to cover ground. There is a term paper to tackle, a chemistry quiz coming up, a patient to interview, some assigned journal articles to read, and a dental appointment at 3 o'clock. But first you'd better throw in a load of laundry (DETOUR). Then the phone rings (DETOUR).

Finally you are off and running. Rounding the first bend, you bump into an old friend who invites you for coffee (DETOUR). Now 2 hours behind schedule, you arrive at the library. Looking for the required journal articles, you happen upon a fascinating issue about career planning (DETOUR). That leaves time to read only three of the required articles before class.

After class, you walk over to the hospital and find that your patient is unavailable. (He is always in physical therapy at this time of day.) Oh well, you can kill some time in the cafeteria (DETOUR).

The patient interview takes longer than you expected, making you 15 minutes late for class. Embarrassed to walk in late, you decide to cut class (DETOUR). You go directly to chem lab and begin preparing for today's assignment.

Leaving lab a few minutes early, you dash to the dentist's office. You are on time, but he isn't. You are kept waiting for an hour. Unfortunately, you left your chemistry notes at the lab, so you decide to write a long-overdue letter to your mom (DETOUR).

With half your face numb, you leave the dentist's office. You drive toward campus intending to start work on that term paper. Caught in rush-hour traffic, you suddenly feel drained. It has been a long day. You deserve an evening off. You turn around and head for home thinking, "There's always tomorrow" (DETOUR).

KNOW THE WARNING SIGNS

The word detour comes from the French meaning "to divert." Diversions come in all shapes, sizes, and disguises. Keeping on course requires constant attention. To avoid unnecessary detours, ask yourself several times a day: "Is what I am doing or about to do helping me reach one of my goals?" If the answer is no, you are on a detour.

Most students who fail to graduate aren't losers; they just get lost. They start out on the right road but forget where they are going. They lose sight of their goal. They are lured off the track by seemingly harmless diversions.

Always keep your eye on the finish line. Never forget that your NUMBER ONE GOAL IS TO GRADUATE.

Goals determine priorities. Priorities determine how you allocate such limited resources as time, money, and energy. Graduation is your long-term goal. All of your short-term goals should contribute directly or indirectly to that end.

The only way to graduate is to stay in school. The only way to stay in school is to successfully complete one test, one paper, one patient, one clinical skill, one term at a time. These are the minor goals that add up to your major goal.

WISHBONES VERSUS BACKBONES

Students spend a lot of time wishing:
"I wish my term paper were done."
"I wish I could lose 10 pounds."
"I wish I didn't procrastinate so much."
"I wish I could get a better grade in chemistry."
"I wish my family helped more with household chores."
"I wish I could get into a different clinical group."

Converting a wish into a goal requires a workable plan. To formulate such a plan, ask yourself the five following questions:

1. What do I need to do to get what I want?
2. What am I willing to do to get what I want?
3. How will getting what I want affect my life?
4. Whom can I count on to help me get what I want?
5. How might I sabotage myself so I don't get what I want?

Let's take "I wish I could get a better grade in chemistry" and work it through from a wish to a goal.

1. *What do I need to do to get a better grade in chemistry?* I might need to do such things as:
   - Spend extra time studying chemistry assignments
   - Memorize formulas
   - Ask questions in class
   - Complete all assignments
   - Join a study group
   - Hire a tutor
   - Buy a study guide or supplementary textbook
   - Change lab partners
   - Ask the instructor for help
   - Do projects for extra credit

2. *What am I willing to do to get a better grade in chemistry?*
   Reading over the list I made in response to the first question, I circle those things I am willing and able to do to improve my grade. I will be scrupulously honest. There is no sense trying to kid myself.
   Knowing what has to be done and doing it are two different things. If I refuse to take the steps I have outlined, getting a better grade in chemistry remains a wish and never becomes a goal.

3. *How will getting a better grade in chemistry affect my life?*
   If I know what I have to do to get a better grade but am unwilling to take the necessary action, this question might

give me the extra incentive I need. The results may be worth the effort if by improving my grade I can keep from flunking out, or raise my GPA, or increase my self-esteem and confidence.

Because I cannot "find" time or "make" time, I am going to have to "take" time away from other activities. Shifting time to chemistry may mean getting up an hour earlier or going to bed an hour later. It may mean spending less time with friends and family. It may mean jeopardizing my grade in another course.

My goals and priorities determine what I will do; they also determine what I will not do.

This is the most difficult aspect of being a goal-oriented student. I am forced to admit that although I may be able to do anything, I simply cannot do everything. The ability to make tough decisions based on goals and priorities is what separates superstudents from so-so students.

4. *Whom can I count on to help me improve my grade in chemistry?*

Me, myself, and I. That's three. Perhaps my instructor, a classmate, my spouse, the lab assistant, or a professional tutor. I will evaluate all possible human resources.

5. *How might I sabotage myself so I don't get a better grade?*

I might give up without even trying. I might continue to cross my fingers, close my eyes, and hope for the best. I might put off taking action until it is too late. I might rationalize by saying I cannot afford to put more time into chemistry, while not admitting that being *unwilling* to pay the price is not the same as being *unable* to pay the price of a higher grade.

By using these five questions, you can establish a plan for achieving any goal: completing a term paper, losing 10 pounds, improving grades, or getting more help around the house. Activating and sticking to the plan takes real backbone.

GOALS TO GO

Goals should be realistic and attainable. Don't become side-tracked by a compulsion for perfection. Some students want not only to graduate but to graduate with honors—or not at all. Settle for pure, unadulterated graduation. Don't take a difficult goal and make it impossible.

Goal-oriented students strive to make everything they do pay off in terms of long-range achievement. They may even take part-time jobs in the health care industry, thinking they will not only earn needed income but will also gain valuable experience.

Instructors advance strong arguments for and against such practice. The "pros" say such jobs provide flexible hours, give students a taste of the real world, boost confidence, and supplement the limited clinical experience provided by the school. The "cons" say such jobs are exhausting and usually pay poorly. The menial jobs offered to students provide meager clinical experience and imprint subordinate status, a mindset that is difficult to break.

Should you take a job in the health care industry while going through nursing school? Again, remember that your goal is to graduate. Choose the job that best contributes to that goal.

If you are thoroughly intimidated by the clinical setting, a hospital job may increase your confidence. As your confidence grows, your performance will improve. On the other hand, if you are floundering academically, stop working altogether or look for a low-stress job that allows time for study, such as being a desk clerk, night watchman, or dispatcher. When choosing your job, be practical. The better the salary, the fewer hours you have to work and the more time you can devote to your education.

Stick to business during business hours. Keep your eye focused on the finish line and you will take fewer detours. Keep evaluating each activity and assignment in terms of your goals. For example, is what you are doing at this very moment contributing to one of your goals? YES. Keep reading!

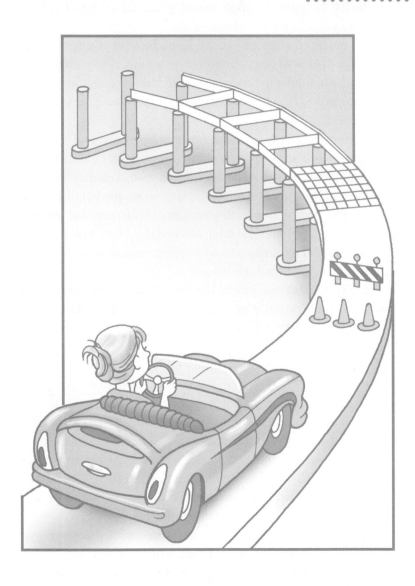

12

You Can't Get There From Here

"A problem is nothing but concentrated opportunity."
—Dr. Norman Vincent Peale

A fter wandering through the New England countryside and becoming hopelessly lost, a motorist stopped and asked a farmer for directions. The farmer paused, then shook his head and replied, "You can't get there from here."

It's an old joke, but the punch line is one that nursing students hear all too often. When you find it necessary to ask for guidance and you are given a you-can't-get-there-from-here answer, don't believe it. Ask again. Ask someone else.

"I wanted to take a business course as an elective, but I didn't have the necessary prerequisite. My advisor suggested I choose something else. Instead, I went to the professor and told him what I hoped to gain from the class and why my life experiences should count as the prerequisite. He granted permission. It was one of the best classes I have ever taken."

Many students make the mistake of asking only one person—often not even the right person. Before you give up, get a second opinion and perhaps a third. Asking for what you want is no guarantee that you will get it, but *not* asking guarantees failure.

A nurse who wanted to work on her bachelor's degree had a list of lower division courses she was required to take before she could proceed. To save money she thought she would take them at the community college instead of the university.

Luckily, her new faculty advisor was a former dean of students. When he interviewed her, he thought attending community college would be a waste of time and money. He encouraged her to make a list of her professional accomplishments, life experiences, and the training sessions she had attended. "Deans read better than they listen," he told her.

She returned to the university with her list in hand. She was immediately placed in upper division courses. Not only did she save thousands of dollars, she saved a year and a half of her life!

If you are going to find your way from one end of nursing to the other, make sure you pack plenty of persistence. If one approach doesn't work, switch to another. Be bold enough to deal directly with the people involved and bright enough to bring concrete evidence.

"One of our instructors talked so fast we could not keep up with her. Several of us asked her to slow down, but within a few minutes she would be spewing forth facts and figures at an incomprehensible rate. Our test scores went down. Finally, we decided to record one of her lectures. We made an appointment and played the tape back to her. After listening she apologized and changed her style. Our test scores improved."

Instructors are not mind readers. If you need help, speak up.

"In one of our courses, 10 different teachers presented material. There was some conflicting information, and as the final exam drew closer, we got very worried. Whom could we trust for the *correct* answer? We asked all the teachers to attend a review session. We asked questions and finally got straight answers."

Faculty members are not purposely insensitive; they are just insanely busy. A major problem for you may look minor on their overcrowded "to do" list. Instead of hoping the instructor will deal with your problem quickly, set a definite time. If you say, "I'll check back with you at 4 o'clock tomorrow," you will be less likely to get lost in the shuffle. When you show up the next day, you will either get your answer or reinforce the urgency of your need. It's better to find out that your problem has been overlooked for 24 hours than for 2 weeks. You may also try sending your instructor an e mail or leaving a phone message or note.

When meeting a problem head on, a good way to rally support is to draft a petition. Follow proper channels and stick to your guns.

"Our library wasn't open on Sundays. We wrote a petition and virtually everyone signed it. The class officers presented it to the dean.

"We were given all sorts of excuses why it couldn't be done. We just kept pushing for it. Like when we were told the budget wouldn't allow it—all sorts of students volunteered to help staff on a rotating basis.

"Finally, they agreed to open for 4 hours on Sunday afternoons. Traffic in the library has been so heavy they are talking about expanding weekend hours next fall."

Complaining is always easier than generating creative alternatives. Before you call attention to a problem, have several possible solutions in mind. In the following situation the students didn't just let off steam, they proposed a way to streamline the system:

"We were required to write out six full nursing-care plans on our patients. Students were staying up so late and coming to clinical so tired they could not function very well.

"We asked the instructors if we could do some of our care plans orally. We figured you have to know your stuff thoroughly either way. The instructors agreed to a trial period. The new system worked so well that both students and instructors voted to keep it going."

In all five of the above examples the students managed to "get there from here." You can be successful, too—*IF* you have the right kind of drive.

PSYCHOLOGY BEHIND THE WHEEL

By now you have noticed that students have very different driving styles. Some are passive. Some are aggressive.

You can always tell passive drivers by the tread marks on their backs. They are quiet, overly cautious, excessively polite, and indecisive. Always waiting to be told what to do and where to go, they create bottlenecks and are a menace to other drivers as well as to themselves.

Aggressive drivers are fast and reckless. They honk once, and if you don't get out of their way, they run right over you. Their hit-and-run techniques leave the nursing course looking like a demolition derby. They don't care who gets hurt as long as they get where they want to go.

Both passive and aggressive students have low self-esteem. Some have none.

As a student you occupy a subordinate role, and most of us have found that "subordinate" is a euphemism for "inferior." Even though you are not inferior, when you occupy the subordinate position, as in parent-child, employer-employee, doctor-nurse, teacher-student, you may begin to have self-doubts. You may feel inferior and behave in inferior ways.

For whatever comfort it is, this problem occurs at all levels of education. Students working on their master's degrees and doctorates experience similar feelings. They begin to question their intelligence and worth. It is just inherent in the role of student.

You don't have to be either passive or aggressive. You can choose a style that is neither reticent nor reckless. You can choose to be *assertive*.

THE ASSERTIVE LANE

Assertiveness is an attitude, coupled with action, that allows you to move through traffic without being injured or injuring others. One way to become more assertive is to adjust your attitude. As your attitude changes, so will your actions.

To offset feelings of inferiority, try viewing your instructors as your employees. After all, you are paying them to teach you the fine art of nursing. They work for you. And, as an employer, you have the right to make requests; ask for improvements; evaluate work performance; and expect loyalty, courtesy, and prompt attention.

An easier way to become more assertive is to adjust your actions. As your behavior changes, so will your attitudes.

How do assertive students act? They stand tall, look you in the eye, and speak up. They are honest enough to express their feelings but tactful enough to protect your dignity. They will laugh with you but never at you. And they love to laugh at themselves.

They are not afraid to say:

"I prefer ..."
"I dislike ..."
"I am concerned ..."
"I need ..."
"I want ..."
"I do not understand ..."
"I disagree ..."
"I expect ..."

Assertive students are able to accept compliments graciously. They are able to accept criticism thoughtfully. When they fail, they look on failure as a learning experience. Then they adjust their course and head off in a new direction.

When faced with tough problems, they look for solutions instead of scapegoats. They are not interested in plotting to get even because they are too busy planning to get ahead. They are not afraid to make decisions and actively pursue their goals.

Basically, assertive students are realists with optimistic overtones. They share common qualities: positive persistence, boldness, and confidence.

Many nursing schools have integrated assertiveness training into the curriculum. On the surface these skills appear so simple that many overlook the potential power of such a tool. Few appreciate the length of time it takes to become proficient with assertiveness: a lifetime.

Passive and aggressive students may survive the nursing curriculum, but only assertive students have the drive to thrive. The same is true of graduate nurses. Only assertive professionals thrive and consistently manage to "get there from here."

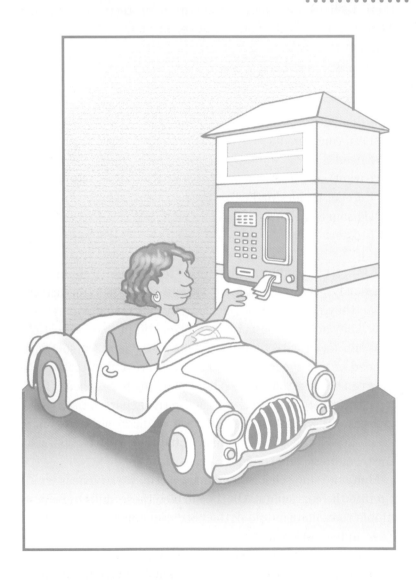

13

Drive-Up Teller

"My memory is so bad, that many times I forget my own name!"
—Cervantes, *Don Quixote*

If you are always in a hurry, you probably like the drive-up window at the bank. You can make transactions without even leaving your car. But you still need to fill out the proper forms. You can't just throw money at the drive-up teller and except it to land in your account.

The same is true of the Memory Bank. You can't just throw information in its general direction and expect to find it later in your account.

The Memory Bank has two branches: short-term and long-term. Cramming is like making a massive deposit in the short-term branch. As long as you withdraw it almost immediately, the lump sum remains intact. If you check on your account a week later, you will find that your deposit has dwindled. A month later you will find a considerable loss. Six months later the account will be closed.

If you want sufficient "funds" available when you go to write state board exams, you cannot rely on your short-term memory bank. The only way to stay solvent is to make deposits in the long-term branch.

The drive-up teller at the long-term branch is best at handling small, regular deposits. Every time you review information, you add to your account. When you review your account, you add interest.

If you tell yourself and others that you have a poor memory, you give your mind permission to forget. Another self-fulfilling prophecy comes true. Instead, tell yourself you have a good or even a great memory. Desire plus confidence pays big dividends.

Some things you think you've forgotten you never actually knew in the first place, such as when you don't quite catch a person's name but you nod and move on.

In the classroom you can't afford to nod and move on. If you don't quite catch the information, ask the instructor to spell the name of the drug or disease. If your notes say there are six common side effects but you can only account for five, ask for the sixth. Get complete, correct information and fix it firmly in your mind.

You cannot remember what you do not understand. One way to check your understanding is to paraphrase the information or think of examples to see whether you really grasp the principles involved.

Information must be meaningful if it is to be remembered. Merging the information with previous or present experiences enables it to be properly catalogued, stored, and retrieved for future use.

When classroom and clinical experiences are synchronized, memory is enhanced. Unfortunately, the two are often out of synch. Only reading about Huntington's chorea simply does not have the same impact as reading about it while caring for a patient with the disease.

MEMORYCISE

Experts often compare memory to a muscle that improves with exercise. Stay in shape; work your memory. Experiment with various techniques such as visualization and mnemonics.

An example of visualization is picturing yourself paddling a microscopic canoe along the bloodstream. Envision passing through each chamber of the heart and navigating the entire system, down to the smallest capillaries. The more vivid or ludicrous the imagery, the more likely you are to remember.

Mnemonics is another key to opening the memory bank. For example, taking the first letter of each word in a series and forming a new word or phrase or a name such as *Roy G. Biv* may help you remember the order of the colors in the rainbow: red, orange, yellow, green, blue, indigo, and violet.

Another way to remember a list of items is to make a sentence using the first letter of every word. Two common ones in the health sciences are (1) "On old Olympus' towering top, a Finn and German viewed a hop" and (2) "Never lower tiny perambulator, mamma might come home." The first sentence helps you remember the twelve cranial nerves (olfactory, optic, oculomotor, trochlear, trigeminal, abducens, facial, acoustic, glossopharyngeal, vagus, accessory, hypoglossal), and the second represents the bones of the wrist (navicular, lunate, triangular, pisiform, multangular/greater, multangular/lesser, capitate, and hamate).

If you want to amass a wealth of information, the following are two ways to make deposits in the Memory Bank.

I. Listening and Learning

To get the most out of the hours you spend in the classroom, follow these five rules: (1) show up, (2) sit in the front, (3) participate in class discussions, (4) ask questions, and (5) look alive! Arrive on time with all necessary equipment. Come rested, nourished, and eager. Choose a seat near the front, away from distractions. Lean forward. Smile. Make eye contact with the instructor. Concentrate. The more you can absorb during class time, the less you will have to absorb on your own time.

Because you are able to hear three times faster than most instructors are able to speak, your mind will have time to wander. Instead of doodling or daydreaming, use that time to organize your notes, differentiate between facts and opinions, fill in gaps, underline material emphasized, and think of practical applications.

During class listen to your inner voice. Are you criticizing the lecturer's ability or appearance? Are you busily refuting or belittling what is being said? When you study under a less-than-ideal instructor, you must make a conscious effort to separate the content from the person presenting it. Avoid running internal arguments or making snide comments to yourself. Listen and learn despite what you think of the instructor.

TAKE NOTES, but don't try to write down every word the instructor says. Few authors and even fewer lecturers are worth quoting verbatim. Before you move your pen, listen. Condense what is said and convert it into your own words. Five minutes of lecture may yield only five words.

Write legibly. Create your own shorthand, but be consistent so that you will be able to decipher it. Here are some abbreviations and symbols that can speed up your note taking and thus give you more time for listening.

♀	female
♂	male
>	greater than
<	less than
=	equals, the same
≠	does not equal, different
×	times
→	leads to, going
←	from, away
↑	up, increasing, above
↓	down, decreasing, under
$	dollar
c̄	with
s̄	without
⊕	positive
⊖	negative
Q.	question
A.	answer
q.	every
∴	therefore
∵	because
~	approximately
Hx	history
Dx	diagnosis
Rx	treatment, prescription

Use this space to write or draw other abbreviations and symbols you frequently use. Compare with classmates.

Make your notes fun to read. Use different colors of paper or ink. Toss in an occasional joke or cartoon.

Some students divide their notebook so that the left-hand page contains text notes and the right-hand page contains class notes. Others prefer separate notebooks for readings and lectures. In either case, leave generous margins where you can make study lists or insert new material.

After class, review your notes as soon as possible. Literally take notes on your notes. Use the margins to summarize. Look for broad principles, see if you understand relationships, separate major from minor facts, assemble any lists worth memorizing, check for discrepancies between lecture and text, and write down questions that occur to you.

II. Reading and Remembering

While reading a journal for nurse educators, an article title caught my eye: "The Relative Influence of Identified Components of Text Anxiety in Baccalaureate Nursing Students." TEXT anxiety? It was a typographical error missed by some proofreader asleep at the switch. The article was on test anxiety, not text anxiety.

But I quickly latched onto the idea. If there isn't a disorder called text anxiety, there should be. For example, adult health nursing textbooks average 2000 pages in length. They will soon have to come equipped with wheels because they're too heavy to carry around. Five years ago, a dozen consultants would be involved in producing a nursing text. Today as many as five dozen experts contribute to each textbook.

If your nursing books appear to be written in a foreign language, they are. They are written in Latin mixed with technical jargon. Instead of skipping over unfamiliar words, flip to the glossary at the back of the text and keep a medical-nursing dictionary close at hand.

Immerse yourself in the language. Study common root words, suffixes, and prefixes. Make flash cards and carry them with you (see Appendix A).

As you struggle to learn this new language, be acutely aware of your feelings and frustrations. Once you begin speaking "Medicalese" like a native, it is easy to forget what patients and their families go through as they struggle to understand us.

As a nursing student you will have not only a horrendous amount of reading but a horrendous amount of hard reading. Educators use a formula based on the length of words and sentences to assess the relative difficulty of written material and assign a grade level to it. For example, the *Reader's Digest* requires grade 8 reading ability, and the *Wall Street Journal* requires grade 10 ability. Nursing students in one baccalaureate program used the formula on their medical-surgical text and found that it required grade 17 ability! When you need 5 years of college to understand a required freshman text, you realize the importance of reading skills.

If you are a poor reader, you will need help sharpening your skills or else you will not survive the nursing curriculum. Ask about programs to improve reading speed and comprehension. Commercial courses are available, but they are usually expensive. Your school may offer a comparable course for much less and may even give you college credit for it.

Here are some tips to help you get more out of your reading time:

Before you begin reading

Pick a place with no distractions, or if you're in your room, padlock the refrigerator, turn off the TV, disconnect the phone, and hang a DO NOT DISTURB sign on the door. Sit at a desk so you can take notes. Choose a chair that is comfortable but not too comfortable. You don't want to doze off. If you need glasses, wear them, and always make sure you have sufficient light.

Ask yourself *why* you are reading this particular material. Consult the chapter objectives if they're provided. Decide whether your mission is to uncover facts, understand principles, answer specific questions, assess relevance, or create a term paper or a research project of your own.

Before reading the first paragraph, take a couple of moments to SKIM the entire chapter or article. To understand what the author considers important, look at section headings, any bold type, italicized words, illustrations, diagrams, charts, or graphs. Read the whole summary. Examine the study questions provided. To understand what your instructor considers important, check the course outline, objectives, study questions, and any handouts pertaining to this assignment.

While you read

Don't just go through the motions. Remember, it's not what you put into reading, it's what you get out of it that counts. The best way to remember what you read is to TAKE NOTES. A much less effective way is to use a highlighter or to underline as you read. Reading by itself is a poor third choice.

Instruct your mind to focus on the material. Watch for connecting words, qualifiers, and punctuation marks that can completely change the meaning. Reread difficult passages slowly. Move your lips. Reading aloud can increase comprehension.

Read to understand, not to memorize. As you take notes, put the material in your own words. If you can put the material in your own words, you understand it. If you understand it, you can remember it.

Vary your speed. (Average reading speed varies from 100 to 400 words per minute.) One of the quickest ways to improve both speed and comprehension is to use your fingertips to "underline" the sentences as you read. A comfortable position is to turn your palm up and use your middle and index fingers. This action pulls your eyes along the page, enabling you to see more words at a time. It also reduces the chances of losing your place or staring at one word while your mind goes elsewhere.

Maintain a positive attitude. Try to keep an open mind. Resist the urge to argue with the author. If you find statements that seem contradictory or confusing, place a question mark in the margin and ask the instructor for clarification.

After reading

Quickly review your notes or scan what you have underlined in the text. Try to sum up the chapter in your own words. Take a second look at any illustrations, charts, or diagrams. Can you explain them without rereading? Can you answer the author's study questions? Your instructor's study questions?

Parking all this information in your long-term memory requires a chemical change to take place in your brain. Excessive physical or emotional activity immediately after a study session can interfere with this process. Instead of going to a football game or fighting with your spouse, put your book under your pillow and sleep on it.

When you check your statement from the long-term memory bank, you will find that you remember every "first" with remarkable clarity—your first patient, your first injection, your first day in surgery. You are also likely to find any information that startled, surprised, amused, or interested you. And you will have total recall of everything your instructor prefaced with, "You don't have to know this for the test but ..." Bank on it!

"We're drowning in information and starving for knowledge."
—Rutherford D. Rogers

"You can never do a kindness too soon, for you never
know how soon it will be too late."
—Ralph Waldo Emerson

"When you get to the end of your rope, tie a knot and hang on."
—Franklin Delano Roosevelt

"If you take too long in deciding what to do with your life,
you'll find you've done it."
—George Bernard Shaw

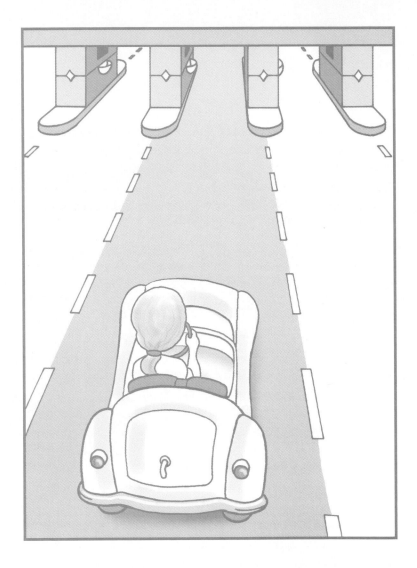

14

Tollbooth

"I have answered three questions, and that is enough."
—Lewis Carroll, *Alice in Wonderland*

Zooming along, you spot a tollbooth. The tollgate is down; the red light is flashing. To go from Aspiring Nurse 101 to Aspiring Nurse 202, you have to come up with the correct change: adequate scores on examinations, finished term papers, evidence of clinical competence, and a suitable GPA.

If you search your pockets and come up short, you may be able to persuade the gatekeeper to let you postpone payment. With an INCOMPLETE in hand you are allowed to "pass."

Don't delude yourself into thinking you can easily make up for lost time on the next leg of the course. Each leg is more difficult than the last, and if you are already pushing hard just to keep up, there will be almost no time for making up.

If you are not seriously ill and no one in the family is dying, it is far better to buckle down and complete this term now. Cut out the frills, get a tutor, burn the midnight oil, forget perfection, and accept a grade that is a notch lower than you'd like. Don't try to carry this term's work into next term.

Testing takes a heavy toll on many students. As test time approaches, they experience headaches, dizziness, diarrhea, insomnia, nausea, and assorted muscle cramps. No amount of studying reduces the panic. During the first few moments of the exam, they literally lose their minds. Everything goes blank.

"I was a babbling nervous wreck, flapping around the room like a wild animal, pouring sweat and unable to concentrate on any

one thought for more than two or three seconds at a time."
—Hunter S. Thompson, *Fear and Loathing in Las Vegas*

Everyone experiences some degree of test anxiety. What may surprise low-performance students is that high-performance students experience the very same physical symptoms, but they instruct their minds not to pay any attention to them. Instead they focus on the test. They quickly become absorbed in the task at hand, and their physical symptoms disappear. High-performance students don't worry about *how* they are doing; they concentrate on *what* they are doing.

If you begin to panic during an exam, close your eyes for a moment. Breathe slowly and deeply. Talk positively to yourself. Knock off the easy questions first. This builds confidence and helps you perform to the best of your ability on the remainder of the test.

If you know a student who suffers from such extreme test anxiety that it would be more properly called "test terror," get him or her professional help.

High-performance students automatically use some simple skills that boost their scores. If you are a student who knows the material as well as your study partners, yet you consistently score lower than they do, these skills can help you even the score.

PREPARATION FOR TESTING

High-performance students find out everything they can about the teacher and the test. First, they study the teacher. Is this instructor bent on helping students succeed or on weeding out as many students as possible? Is this a person obsessed with trivia or one who concentrates on principles, ideas, and relationships? What are this person's special interests and areas of expertise?

Second, they gather all the information they can about the test. What kind of test will it be? Multiple-choice or essay? What material will be covered? Text and lecture only, or other reading assignments and laboratory work as well?

The best source of information on the test is the teacher. Just ask! Most are perfectly willing to share this information. You may also find it helpful to ask former students.

An excellent way to prepare for a new test is to study an old one. You may be surprised to learn that many instructors leave copies of their old tests on file at the library or in the department office. Even if the instructor has changed, chances are the course content hasn't. Many questions will be reworded but recognizable.

Believe it or not, you are better off with a teacher who gives frequent tests and quizzes. If there are only two tests given all term, too much is riding on each. By the time you figure out the teacher's style, it is almost too late to improve your grade. If you have a teacher who skimps on tests, it becomes even more important to track down everything possible about the exam beforehand.

When is the best time to begin studying for exams? The first day of class. Successful students attend class religiously, listen intently, take careful notes, and mark information the instructor emphasizes for special study. Soon after each class, they condense their notes and review them frequently. (For more study tips see Chapter 10, "More Miles Per Gallon.")

Begin studying for a specific test 2 or 3 weeks in advance. Remember these words: READ * WRITE * REVIEW * RECITE. As you *read, write*! Don't just underline. Jot down the main facts, names, dates, ideas, and relationships. Put everything in your own words. If you can do that, you understand it. If you understand it, you can remember it. *Review* what you've written. Condense your notes. Reread them as often as possible. Close your text or notebook and *recite* what you have learned.

Most students find it helpful to study for tests with a partner or a small group. You often discover things you may have overlooked or underemphasized. When you coach other students, you get a better grasp of the material yourself.

Some major tests are not given in the regular classroom. Find out where the test will be given. Visit the room and actually spend time studying there. The more comfortable you are in the test room, the more relaxed you will be and the better you will perform.

Twenty-Four Hours Before the Test

Keep food intake and exercise on the light side. Lay out equipment you want to take with you: pens, pencils, erasers, scratch paper, blue books, calculator, wristwatch, sweater, and—if it is a long test—a snack such as candy, peanuts, or raisins.

Surround yourself with pleasant, positive people. Avoid situations that depress or aggravate you.

Ten Minutes Before the Test

Arrive at the test site 10 minutes before the exam. That's enough time to relax and not enough time to panic. Choose a seat away from windows, doors, aisles, friends, and enemies. If you are left-handed, make sure you get a left-handed desk.

Breathe slowly and deeply. Tense and relax your muscles, especially those in your neck and shoulders. Give yourself a pep talk, not an ultimatum.

During the Test

Listen carefully to oral instructions. Ask for clarification if you are confused. Read written instructions carefully. Take time to work through any sample questions provided. It will save you time in the long run.

Skim the entire test. How many questions are there? How much time can you allow for each? Are the questions weighted differently? For example, 100 multiple-choice questions may be worth only 40% of the grade, the matching section worth 10%, and the two essay questions worth 50%. Divide your time accordingly.

If marking on the test is allowed, scribble things you are afraid you will forget—names, dates, formulas, principles—on one of the corners. Circle or underline key words and phrases in the instructions. Examine the stem of each question for significant phrases such as "same as," "opposite of," or "only one."

Work quickly. Leave the toughies and time wasters for last. Remember that many answers are found or alluded to in other questions. Keep your eyes open.

A word of caution: because you will be skipping over some questions, periodically check to make sure the number on the question and the number on the answer sheet match.

Tips for MULTIPLE-CHOICE Items

- Read directions carefully.
- Work quickly. Put a star or checkmark by questions you want to return to later if you have time.
- Formulate your own answer before you read the answers given.
- Read every given answer.
- Eliminate implausible answers.
- Watch for absolutes and qualifiers. Answers containing "always," "never," "all," or "none" are usually incorrect.
- In many nursing exams multiple-choice questions will be related to rather lengthy case studies. To avoid delays caused by rereading, scan all questions *before* reading the case study. Then your eyes will be more attuned to the important information.

Tips for TRUE-FALSE Items

- The longer the true-false statement, the more likely it is to be TRUE.
- There are usually more TRUE statements because they are easier to write.
- Most statements come verbatim from text or lecture. If it looks familiar, play your hunch.
- Statements containing "all," "only," "always," or "because" are usually FALSE.
- Statements containing "none," "generally," or "usually" are more often TRUE.
- If the statement is long or complicated, break it into smaller parts. Remember, if one part is false, the whole statement is FALSE.

- Don't change answers. On true-false items your first impression is usually correct.

Tips for MATCHING Items

- Check to see whether answers are used only once or more than once.
- Do easy matches first.
- Work down the column with the longest phrases.
- Look for patterns: dates-events, terms-definitions, people-contributions.

Tips for SHORT ANSWER and FILL-IN-THE-BLANK Items

- Look for clues in language and sentence construction.
- The length of the blank usually indicates the length of the answer desired.
- If you know two possible answers, give both. You will rarely be penalized, and you may get extra credit.
- Make an educated guess. Don't leave the blankety-blank blank.

Tips for MATHEMATICAL Items

- Read each question very carefully. Write down the givens, what you are expected to find, and any formulas you plan to use.
- Estimate the answer before doing calculations so you'll know whether you're close or far afield.
- Write legibly, and keep numbers in distinct columns.
- Copy accurately.
- Check units of measure—ounces, drams, millimeters.
- Use a calculator and any other helps permitted.
- If abstractions confuse you, substitute simple numbers for symbols.
- Check math by working the problem backwards.
- If the answer is in multiple-choice form and you haven't the foggiest idea, you can usually eliminate the highest and lowest answers given.

Tips for ESSAY Items

- When you are offered a choice of essay questions, read all of them before deciding which to tackle.
- Beside each question, quickly list the facts and ideas that pop into your head.
- Budget your time. Spend 50% outlining the answer and 50% writing it.
- Know who will be grading the exam. If it will be scored by a teaching assistant, forgo fancy writing and stuff every name, date, fact, idea, and key phrase you can remember into the answer.
- Underline key words in directions. Know precisely what you are to do. For example:

Summarize

Means to give a concise review of the main ideas.

Explain

Means to give the how or why of something.

Illustrate

Means to give effective examples.

Discuss

Means to explain and elaborate.

Define

Means to explain the meaning.

List

Means to give a series of items or ideas without elaborating.

Outline

Means to write only main ideas or facts.

Compare

Means to show similarities.

Contrast

Means to show differences.

- Organize your essay: title, topic sentence, main body, and conclusion.
- Make a final check for mechanics and spelling if time permits.
- If you run out of time, write "I ran out of time. Please accept my outline." You will get partial credit, and you may even get full credit.

Questionable Items

- If you are totally confused, don't panic. Ask the test monitor for clarification.
- Don't let toughies derail you. Move on to the next question. Your unconscious mind will go to work on the tough one while your conscious mind works on the next one. Something in another question may jog your memory or clear up confusion.
- Break long, complicated questions into small, manageable parts. Read slowly, moving your lips or subvocalizing each word.
- If two answers seem correct, choose the more obvious.
- If no answer looks correct, choose the most nearly correct answer.
- Give the answer the instructor wants. Don't quibble!
- Always *guess* unless there is a penalty for guessing (i.e., more points are subtracted for giving a wrong answer than for giving no answer), in which case, play the odds.
- If you wish to protest an item, see the instructor after the test but before grades are given out.

Just Before Turning in Your Test

- Erase all stray marks on the answer sheet.
- Make sure that your name is on each sheet.
- Reread directions.
- Look at any questions you have flagged for further consideration. If you honestly believe an answer should be changed, change it. You will probably be correct. Just don't waffle back and forth and back again.
- Fill in all the blanks.
- Use all the time available.
- Never give up.

FINAL TOLLBOOTH: STATE BOARD EXAMS

Taking some college courses is like being vaccinated. Once you've given it a shot and passed, you are "immune." Even if you can't remember anything from the course 2 weeks after the final, you never have to take the course again. For courses like that you can cram. In 3 days you can learn everything you need to pass the course, and 3 days later you can forget it all.

Nursing isn't like that. You will not only be required to remember, you will be required to understand virtually everything from your basic nursing courses. You will be expected to build on that information in more advanced courses, and every day you will apply what you've learned as you care for patients. The study of nursing demands continuous review. There is no way to cram and survive.

Even after you have successfully completed all your schooling, there is still one final exam standing between you and your license to practice nursing. Although everyone reviews for state boards, no one can cram. That's why the best time to begin studying for the state board exams is the first day—and every day—of class.

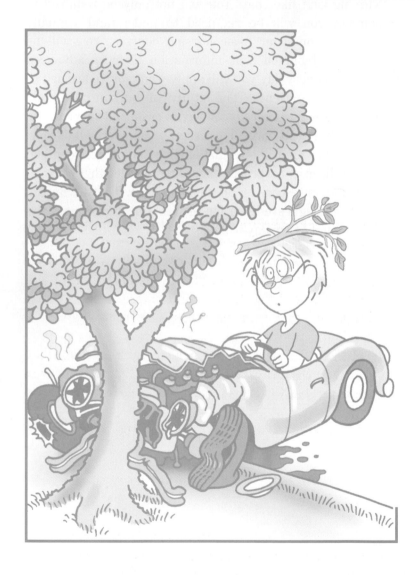

Totaled

"I failed! Now I'll never be a nurse!"

Hold on. Before you declare yourself a total wreck, take a closer look at the damage. You may not require a tow truck. You may just need some emergency road service.

If you've flunked an exam, bombed on a term paper, been chewed out by an instructor, or had an irate patient demand to see a "real" nurse, it can be devastating, but it is far from fatal.

Most failures signal a need for change, not an end to all your career aspirations. A poor performance in the classroom or clinical area warns you that things are not going as they should. Heed the warning.

The first step is to determine exactly what happened. Is this an isolated incident or a symptom of an underlying problem? Occasionally, failure is due to circumstances beyond your control. *Occasionally.*

To fail has several different meanings. For example, to fail means:

- To lose strength; to fade away or die away; to stop functioning
- To fall short
- To become absent or inadequate, to be deficient
- To disappoint the expectations or trust of someone

Let's look at how each of these meanings applies to the most common reasons for student failure and explore possible remedies.

"To Lose Strength, to Fade Away or Die Away, to Stop Functioning"

Lack of commitment

Lack of commitment is the number one reason for failure. Becoming a nurse is not a driving passion. Either you have temporarily lost sight of your goal or you have changed goals—consciously or unconsciously. Your interest is waning. You don't really hate nursing, but you don't really love it. You are lukewarm, and it is beginning to show in your grades.

Remedy: Everyone has a slump now and then. You may need a good night's sleep, a vitamin supplement, a day by the seashore, or a pep talk from a nurse who loves her work. For lingering slumps, talk with your advisor or a guidance counselor. It may be wise to voluntarily step out of school for a while rather than have failure make your exit mandatory.

Laziness

Becoming a nurse is requiring a lot more work than you ever imagined. Frankly, you can't summon up the vim, vigor, and vitality required to keep pace with the rest of the class.

Remedy: Shove it in gear or start looking for a less demanding way to make a living.

Illness

Sudden illness in yourself or a family member can throw a monkey wrench in the best-laid plans. Student nurses are on such an "unforgiving" time schedule that a few days out of commission can spell disaster.

Remedy: If the interruption is brief and you can get up to speed quickly, you may be able to catch up and finish the term successfully. If not, negotiate with the individual instructors for an "Incomplete" or an alternate assignment. Talk with your advisor about all the options. Check on the school's policy regarding withdrawal without penalty. Before you take the off ramp, make sure there is an on ramp available. Once off the track, you may be out of the course for a year or more.

"To Fall Short"

Lack of ability

Caring *about* sick people is one thing; caring *for* them is quite another. Nursing demands peak performance physically, mentally, and emotionally. You may be intellectually gifted but a basket case emotionally. You may be emotionally strong but physically frail. Not everyone has the right mix of talents, skills, and abilities to make a success of nursing.

Remedy: Determine which limitation is causing the failure. You can shore up sagging abilities, but it may require an inordinate amount of time and energy. Decide whether you are both willing and able to take the corrective action. Seek professional counsel.

Self-defeating behaviors

Self-defeating behaviors might be more accurately called "imagined lack of ability." If you expect to fail, you will rarely be disappointed. Pessimists, nitpickers, worrywarts, perfectionists, and procrastinators are some who fit into this category.

Remedy: Sometimes just recognizing a self-defeating behavior can change its impact so dramatically that you can convert failure into success. Other times, these behaviors are so entrenched that professional help is required to overcome their crippling effects.

"To Become Absent or Inadequate, To Be Deficient"

Absenteeism

When Woody Allen was asked the secret of his success, he quipped that showing up was 80%. Students who fail are those who fail to show up for class. Grades are directly correlated with class attendance.

Remedy: Force yourself to attend every class. Sit near the front.

Poor study habits

College students have to run full speed just to keep up. If your study skills are not up to snuff, your workload will be doubled. Not only will you have to master the subject matter, you will have to master study skills as well. By the time you realize the importance of being efficient and effective in your study habits, it may be too late. The damage will be done.

Remedy: *Habit* is the key word. Habitual study. Consistently putting in time with the books is vital if you are to survive. Knowing how to get the most out of your study time will help you thrive. For extra help, see Chapters 10, 13, 14, and 23.

Outside activities

Although outside activities can greatly enrich your life, an overdose can kill you. The famous last words of many former students who failed to graduate are, "Never let school interfere with your education."

You may be a first-time-away-from-home student who is intoxicated by your new freedom. You are so busy experiencing life that you haven't had time to think about grades. Or you may be a superstudent, who edits the school paper, serves as council president, builds the homecoming float, and works 20 hours a week as a clerk. Or you may be the midlife mother-wife, promising that nothing will change just because you've added being a student to your already busy schedule. You still manage to keep the house spotless, teach Sunday school, manage the charity bazaar, and turn out gourmet meals when entertaining.

The only thing wrong with outside activities is that they gobble up time, and time is an irreplaceable resource. An A in homecoming, parenting, or partying will not balance an F in anatomy, microbiology, or organic chemistry.

Remedy: Recognize that to succeed as a student you will have to limit outside activities for a few years. Reevaluate the people, events, and things in your life. Simplify, simplify, simplify. Stick with a couple of the most satisfying activities, and slough off everything else.

"To Disappoint the Expectations or Trust of Someone"

Perhaps the most difficult aspect of failure is having to face all those people who expected you to become a nurse. Your parent or spouse says, "I don't understand. Why are you dropping out? You've wanted to be a nurse since you were 6 years old."

What do you say to people like that? First, remind them that you aren't 6 years old anymore, and suggest that no one should be bound by career choices made in childhood. "Yes, I always dreamed of being a nurse, but now I'm awake. And when I looked at nursing with my eyes wide open, I realized it wasn't the career for me."

Some things are more attractive from a distance, such as a beautiful suit that catches your eye from clear across the store. It looks great on the hanger, but when you try it on it just doesn't fit.

You've tried on nursing. It doesn't fit. Minor alterations are always possible, but major alterations may be impossible—or at the very least, impractical.

Remedy: Whether you failed nursing or nursing failed you, give yourself time to grieve. Loss is always painful, even if it is only a dream that has died. Then get out and shop around for a career that does fit. Someday when you are a successful lawyer, architect, teacher, mechanic, musician, or florist, a nurse will walk by and you'll say with a sigh, "There but for the grace of God (and a few lousy grades) go I."

• • •

A nursing professor is currently serving on a board of directors with a former student to whom she gave a failing grade in a leadership course years before. In retrospect, the professor attributes the failure to her own inexperience as a teacher at the time and the student's nonconformity, which was misinterpreted by the faculty.

Today that former student is not only a nurse but heads a multimillion dollar company. And she failed LEADERSHIP!

Neither has mentioned the incident, and frankly, it is driving the professor nuts. I suggested she take her former student to lunch and have a good laugh over it. That failure may have been the catalyst that drove the student to success. After all, the best revenge is living well.

"Defeat may serve as well as victory to shake the soul and let the glory out."
—Senator Sam J. Ervin, Jr.

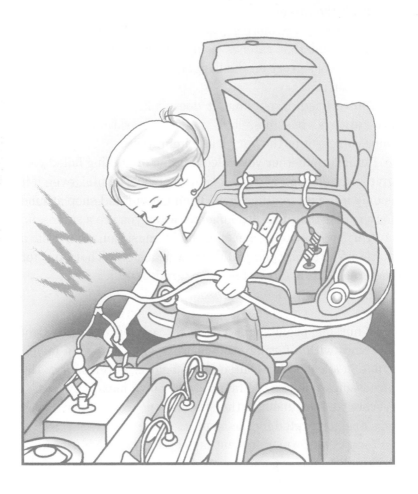

16

How to Jump-Start Your Battery

"The tougher you are on yourself, the easier life will be on you."
—Zig Ziglar

Have you ever jumped into your car and found the battery dead as a doornail? If you were parked on a hill, you may have tried this simple trick: you let the car start rolling, popped the clutch, and the engine leaped to life.

Sometimes you jump into a term paper and find it dead as a doornail. You sit at the computer, fingers poised, but nothing happens. The words won't come.

Instead of sitting immobilized for lack of the *right* words, type *any* words: random thoughts, sentence fragments, even gibberish. Don't waste time agonizing over the opening paragraph; skip to the middle section. Begin anywhere you can. Get rolling, pop the clutch, and your engine will leap to life. Remember, it is easier to steer a moving vehicle, and it is easier to edit than to write.

Have you ever found yourself reading the same sentence for the third time? That's a sure sign your battery is dead. You need to recharge before you continue. Get up and splash some cool water on your face. Stretch. Reach for the ceiling, then bend over and touch your toes. Do a dozen jumping jacks. Then sit down and begin reading again.

Does this sound familiar? "I know I *should* work on my care plan, but I just don't *feel* like it right now." Forget feelings. MOVE! Put the machinery in motion, and the *feeling* will follow.

If you are sitting idle alongside the road, here is one way to jump-start your battery. Take your kitchen timer and set it for 5 minutes. Pick up that required reading, your research notes, or the care plan you have to do, and agree to work on it for just 5 minutes. You can stand anything for 5 minutes, right?

In that few moments something miraculous usually happens. The most inert students are energized. When the timer rings, odds are you will continue the activity. You won't even want to quit.

Another way to conquer procrastination is to make an appointment with yourself. Select a definite day, time, and place to begin working on a project. Keep that appointment.

THE PSYCHOLOGY OF PUTTING IT OFF

Almost every student procrastinates. Some do it because they are rebellious. They hate being told what to do and when to do it. By refusing to meet deadlines, they experience a temporary high and a fleeting feeling of being in charge.

Others are thrill seekers. They see the deadline as the edge of a cliff. Driving pell-mell, they see how close they can come to the edge before chickening out. At the last minute, they veer off and hurriedly do the project.

Some students love to experiment. They want to see whether the instructor really means *DEAD*line or whether special privileges will be granted to keep them from a fatal plunge.

Still others use procrastination to protect their fragile egos. Endorsing the "I-work-better-under-pressure" theory, they try to cram 2 weeks of work into 2 days. In the last few hours they exert superhuman effort. If the project fares well, it affirms their better-under-pressure theory. If the project fares poorly, they comfort themselves with the thought that they could have done better. There just wasn't enough time. Afraid to really put their ability to the test, they continue to procrastinate. After all, wouldn't it be mortifying to work all term and produce only a mediocre project?

OUT OF NEUTRAL AND INTO GEAR

If you are struggling to overcome procrastination, here is another gimmick to help you get moving. Take a piece of paper and fold it in half. On the right-hand side, list everything you have to gain by completing a project on time or ahead of schedule. On the left-hand side, list everything you have to gain by putting the project off until the last possible moment.

If you are honest, you will have to admit that the only things gained by procrastination are anxiety, guilt, low grades, and other assorted headaches. If you tackle projects promptly and aim for early completion, your grades will rise along with your self-confidence and self-esteem. You will experience relief, joy, a sense of accomplishment, and a certain amount of smugness. You will be able to take time off for good behavior and really enjoy yourself.

Time off is one thing procrastinators actually don't have. Undone work, unmet deadlines, and the dread of facing irate instructors haunt their leisure hours. Every time they pass the library or glance at their dusty keyboards, they suffer pangs of guilt. Constantly nagged by the thought of what they *should* be doing, they find it almost impossible to relax.

If you are a particularly stubborn procrastinator, you may have to use the carrot-and-stick approach. This method moves stubborn students as well as stubborn mules. For example, to get students moving, instructors dangle "carrots" in front of them, such as smiles, praise, recognition, good grades, merit scholarships, a spot on the dean's list, and opportunities for choice assignments. For "sticks" they use frowns, criticism, harassment, low grades, probation, and failure.

Some students respond more quickly to carrots; others, to sticks. How about you?

To get yourself moving, you can devise your own system of rewards and punishments. When you keep regular study hours or perform assignments promptly, reward yourself. Take a bubble bath, have lunch with a friend, watch your favorite TV program, have a cup of gourmet coffee, read the next chapter in a bestseller. If you fail to keep regular study hours or to meet a deadline, punish yourself. Take a cold shower, unplug the TV set, go without coffee, do a chore you despise, eat a bologna-banana sandwich.

To be most effective, your reward and punishment system must be highly individualized. One student's reward is another's punishment. Create your own list (see p. 107).

Just like this list, batteries have both positive and negative poles. Whenever you need a jump-start, use one of your carrots, one of your sticks, or a combination of the two.

Check your battery frequently. If you begin to feel run down, recharge by taking a different route home, eating supper at breakfast time, sending yourself roses, watching a vintage movie, wading in a brook, or diving into a new adventure.

Don't forget that batteries also run down when you turn off your engine but leave your lights on. Turn off your lights. Get some sleep.

CARROTS	STICKS
People, places, things, and activities I enjoy	People, places, things, and activities I dislike

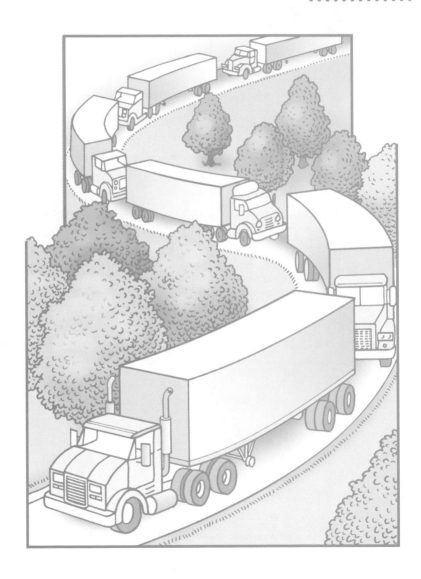

17

10-4, Good Buddy

"All for one, one for all, that is our device."
—Alexandre Dumas, *The Three Musketeers*

*L*ong, lonely stretches of road loom between you and graduation. No one can possibly know the trials and tribulations you are going through. No one except *another nursing student*. That's why the best way to keep on truckin' is to form a convoy.

In a project sponsored by the University of San Francisco to help retain freshman nursing students, faculty members were surprised to learn how much homesickness was a factor in a student's decision to leave school. The first couple of months are the hardest. This is especially true for students who can't get home on weekends because of time, distance, or money problems. To curb the impact of homesickness, the project members suggested linking lonely students together, sponsoring group activities on weekends, or having a local student invite a stranded student home with him or her. Just letting the homesick students know that what they were feeling was normal and temporary helped a lot.

Some of their other suggestions to help freshman nursing students survive included having group and individual counseling sessions, having an intensive orientation program to help students sharpen their study skills and time management abilities, getting the new students involved with upperclassmen in the nursing school, encouraging participation in fun activities as well as study groups, and assisting them with personal problems as well as academic difficulties.

Marc Fisher, a columnist for the *Washington Post*, wrote about how the city government had planted 21 trees in his neighborhood and 6 months later all had died. In contrast, he told about a nearby neighborhood where 120 trees had been planted at the same time. All were alive and well. What made the difference?

One woman. Her name is Penny Moser. She attached a plastic pouch to each of the 120 trees with a note that said, "Hello, I'm your new tree. Please could you adopt me?" Inside the pouch was an information sheet that explained that to survive the first year, the tree needed to be watered at least once a week. Most of the trees were quickly adopted as people signed up to be the "foster parents." Even the "orphans" were watered regularly.

To survive the first year, students need to be watered and nourished. Some schools do a better job of that than others. At Catholic University in Washington, DC, former dean, Ann Marie Brooks, enlisted alumni to adopt students. Each student was paired with a sponsor/mentor who was to follow him or her through the whole 4 years. Maybe she should have had them wear signs saying, "Hello, I'm your new nursing student. Please could you adopt me?"

If you are ever feeling lonely and overwhelmed, you might enjoy this wonderful Emily Dickinson poem titled "I'm Nobody! Who Are You?":

I'm Nobody! Who are you?
Are you—Nobody—Too?
Then there's a pair of us?
Don't tell! They'd advertise—you know!
How dreary—to be—Somebody!
How public—like a Frog—
To tell one's name—the livelong June—
To an admiring Bog!

Nursing students often band together to survive. Without the buddy system, many simply would not make it. When you have to drive in the dark as much as nursing students do, it's reassuring to hear a friendly voice and know you are not alone. Even though you know you must haul your own load, the trip is safer and more enjoyable when you share the road with others.

SAFETY IN NUMBERS

Traveling with a group reassures you that you are on the right road. Just knowing you are not alone keeps panic at a manageable level. As you exchange ideas and experiences, your confidence grows.

The group helps you clear up mysteries, distinguish facts from rumors, set priorities, and achieve goals. Good buddies not only cheer you up when you are losing, they cheer you on when you are winning.

Belonging to a group has several other advantages:

- Working together facilitates problem solving.

"I am in a support group consisting of older students with children. We were all frantically trying to keep our stress levels down and our time-management skills up. After we formed the group, we found we could help each other solve problems on the home front as well as in the classroom. We encourage each other to take 1 day at a time, to prioritize, to do only what needs to be done, and not to hesitate to ask for help—at home or in school."

- Camaraderie replaces competition.

"Joining a study group was the best thing I ever did. I learned to compete with myself, not with other students."

- Group membership fosters cooperation.

"Instead of every student carrying a whole satchel of books to the clinical area, each student in our group carries a different one. That way all of our books are available for reference, but no one gets a broken back. Besides, there's not enough room in the clinical area to store any more of those 40-pound books!"

- Studying with a group means less chance of overlooking or missing important material.

"Our instructors all talk so fast that I knew I was missing things that were important. In study group I spend a few moments comparing my notes with classmates' notes. That way I can fill in the blank spots. My grades have really improved since I started studying with a group."

STRENGTH IN NUMBERS

If you're on your own, you may hesitate to challenge a school policy, call the instructor's attention to inconsistencies, or make special requests. Group support can give you courage.

"We were faced with so much material for each test that we were overwhelmed. We approached the instructors and told them we wanted to have four tests instead of two. And they went for it!"

Studying with friends can lift not only your spirits, but also your GPA.

"I was disappointed in my grade in micro. I thought I had a 'B' going for me, but I received a 'C'. When I mentioned it in my study group, they insisted I talk with the instructor and report back. I did get a 'B'! (There was a computer error.) Without group support and encouragement, I would never have approached the instructor."

Groups can decrease depression and increase productivity.

"Our class was always bitching and complaining about the heavy workload, the tedious assignments, etc. Some of us decided to form a study group with one rule: 'No Bitching.' Instead of complaining about tiresome assignments, we figure out ways to do them better and faster than if we tried to do them alone. We make lists, cross out days on the calendar, and generally encourage each other to think positively. Things still aren't perfect, but we're a lot less depressed."

If you aren't already in a study group, shop around for one. If you can't find one, start one. If you're hesitant, just try it out and see how you like it. For example, organize a temporary group to prepare for one event, such as a major exam or a massive project. If you like studying and working together, you can meet on a more permanent basis.

Your schedule is most likely to mesh with those of other students in your clinical rotation. See if you can interest a half dozen of them in joining you.

Successful study groups have certain ground rules. For the group to be effective, every nursing student in it must agree to the following.

SUCCESSFUL STUDY GROUPS

1. Understand and accept the purpose or mission.
2. Contribute ideas, information, opinions, and feelings.
3. Invite and encourage other members to do the same.
4. Listen intently.
5. Demonstrate respect and support for other members.
6. Help keep the discussion relevant.
7. Periodically help summarize the major points.
8. Give examples and share pertinent clinical experiences.
9. Recognize conflict and controversy as potentially positive, and refuse to see it as a personal rejection.
10. Refrain from eating, smoking, or *knitting* during the session.

HOW TO MAKE A GOOD STUDY GROUP BETTER

Time
Always meet at the same time.

Place
Always meet at the same place.

Begin
Always begin on time.

Monitor
Appoint a monitor to keep the group on target and the discussion moving. Focus on the here and now. Don't let the group spend too much time dwelling in the past or fretting about the future.

Goal
At the beginning of the session, state the goal. "Today we will discuss Chapters 4 and 5," or "This group is reviewing for the anatomy midterm."

Discuss
Allow free-flowing discussion of anything relevant to the group's goal. Identify major concepts, clarify discrepancies between text and lecture, share examples from clinical experience, relate theory to practice. If questions arise that cannot be quickly and accurately answered, don't waste time pooling ignorance. Appoint one member to check with the instructor and report back to the group.

Review
Review lecture notes, highlights of outside readings, films, class objectives, lists to be memorized, etc.

Quiz
Drill each other. Use test questions at the end of the chapter or, better yet, construct your own.

"Lately we've each been bringing two 'trivia' questions to group. It's not only fun, it also forces each member to read and review before the study session. Constructing questions has helped me think the way instructors think when they're making up tests."

Summarize
Periodically pause and recap the major points under discussion. At the end of the session, summarize what you have accomplished and list the things that still need to be done.

Divide
Whenever possible, divide tasks and activities.

"We split up the objectives, with each member being responsible for just a few. That person gathers the information and brings copies for everyone to the next meeting. It saves so much time!"

Assign
Assign individuals or subgroups to tasks, and be sure to specify dates for completion.

End
Always end on time.

Socialize
After the official end of the group, members may feel free to leave or to stay and chat. The benefits of playing together should not be underestimated.

"We had a problem maintaining student morale, so about once a month we have some kind of a get-together where we can relax and talk or joke about our problems. Last semester we had three hours between classes, and every so often we'd order pizza to be brought in or we'd go out for lunch. At our Christmas party we all got together and composed a letter to Santa telling him about all our 'goofs' in clinical. It was fun and reassuring to hear that everyone else made 'goofs' like I did."

When students form study groups or support groups, they are "networking." You may be interested to learn that student networks reach far beyond your own campus. They operate on a national and an international level. If you would like to extend your network, write to:

National Student Nurses' Association
455 Main Street, Suite 606
Brooklyn, NY 11202
http://www.nsna.org
or
Canadian Nursing Students Association
325-350 Albert Street
Ottawa, Ontario, Canada K1R 181
http://www.cnsa.ca

Registered nurses band together in groups for the same reason students do—to survive. And for one even better reason—to thrive! If you would like more information about networks available for registered nurses, see Appendixes E and F for the names and addresses of major nursing associations.

Students helping students. Nurses helping nurses. That's a 10-4, Good Buddy.

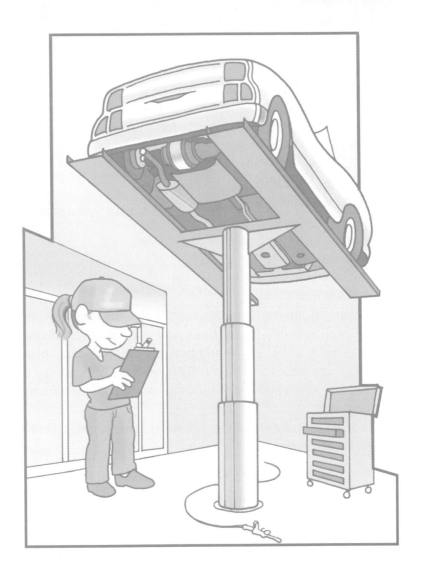

Preventive Maintenance

If you are a smart driver, you know the value of preventive maintenance. You take simple actions to stop problems before they start. You know that by investing a few minutes, you can add years to the life of your car.

Every time you turn the key in the ignition, you should watch for warning lights on the dashboard. When you stop for gasoline, you should check the oil, water, and air pressure in the tires. Every few thousand miles, you should change the oil in your car, and after several thousand miles, you should replace the spark plugs and examine the fan belt for wear.

SELF-SERVICE

In fact, you may take better care of your car than you do of yourself. Those of us attracted to the helping professions are often good at taking care of everyone's needs but our own. We talk a lot about high-level wellness, stress management, and self-actualization; but few of us apply these concepts to our own lives.

We wouldn't run our machinery into the ground, but our personal motto seems to be "Don't stop till you drop." We don't even take time to fuel properly. We skip breakfast, eat lunch out of a vending machine, and drive through "Burgers R Us" for dinner.

Isn't it a pity that nursing students don't come equipped with instrument panels? Then you would know at a glance if your engine was overheating or your brake fluid was running low. Unfortunately, you have no gauges, bells, whistles, or warning lights. Before you realize it, you may drive yourself right into a breakdown.

Preventive maintenance for humans is not as clear-cut as it is for vehicles. It probably includes things such as the following:

- Exercising regularly
- Reducing caffeine
- Avoiding unproductive stress
- Eliminating tobacco and alcohol
- Getting sufficient rest
- Taking vitamin supplements
- Keeping your sense of humor

The key words for a healthy lifestyle are *balance* and *moderation.*

When you find yourself under a lot of pressure and you need to talk things out, you may not be able to find a sympathetic ear. Instead of mumbling to yourself, you may find it helpful to keep a written journal, a daily diary of everything that happens to you as a nursing student. For some reason, talking to yourself on paper is considered sophisticated. Talking to yourself out loud is considered schizophrenic.

Writing allows you to vent feelings safely, unscramble puzzling situations, explore new insights, and put events in perspective. Like a good friend, the journal "remembers" everything you've been through: all the firsts, all the good times, all the adventures and misadventures. On a bad day, when you forget how far you've come, the journal reminds you of your triumphs, not just your tragedies. The journal documents your growth. It chronicles not only your life and times but also the times of your life.

You can purchase an elegantly bound book full of blank pages or use a loose-leaf binder and ordinary notepaper. The journal is for your eyes only. There is no need to worry about spelling, punctuation, or grammar. You may worry about those things later if you decide to convert it to a bestseller.

Every so often, take a quick read of your daily journals. If the same problems and worries keep cropping up, you could be headed for depression. Researchers at the University of Michigan call it "rumination." Psychologist Susan Nolen-Hoeksema says women are prone to brood over problems instead of solving them and moving on with their lives.

Rumination may explain why women are twice as likely as men to fall victim to depression. Women experience more chronic strain than men, and they tend to feel less mastery and control over their lives. They ruminate. That aggravates the chronic strain, accentuates the lack of mastery and control, and increases the rumination. It's a vicious cycle. And the bad news is that bitching doesn't help.

What can you do? Watch yourself. Identify problems. Solve them. Don't get sucked into the downward spiral.

In the words of Mother Goose:

For every evil under the sun
There is a remedy or there's none.
If there is one, try and find it.
If there isn't, never mind it.

Being a nursing student can throw everything out of kilter. So pamper yourself. Have regular checkups. Use common sense. And WEAR SUPPORT HOSE! Remember, it is easier to prevent problems than to correct them.

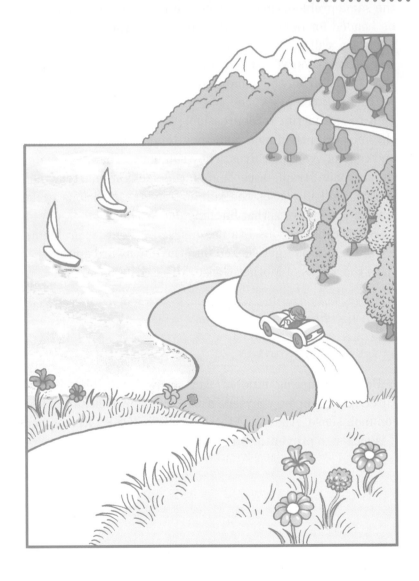

19

Scenic Routes

"A university must give its priority to the numerically small but historically significant band of men and women who believe the worth and dignity of knowledge does not depend solely upon its current usefulness."
—Kingman Brewster

As a nursing student you are usually compelled to go for speed and distance. The only chance you have to leave the main highway is through an occasional elective.

When it comes to choosing an elective, be sure to take the scenic route. Get as far away from nursing as possible. A brief excursion to some out-of-the-way discipline can be thoroughly refreshing and can help you return to the hard, fast pace of nursing with renewed energy and unusual insights.

Watch out for what former University of Rochester President Dennis O'Brien calls the "careerist syndrome." Having a rigid, narrow focus on career goals means missing exciting educational opportunities and graduating ill-equipped to deal with a fast-changing, increasingly complex world.

Once in a while, you need a reminder that the whole world does not revolve around science or sickness. There are other worlds: art, music, drama, politics, economics, business, architecture ... agriculture! Use your electives for field trips to these other worlds.

Nursing requires you to be so perfect and so practical that you may need an elective that allows you to be imperfect and impractical. Use electives for mental health breaks.

Because advisors are paid to look out for your future, they sometimes overlook your present. Consider your advisor's list of should-and-ought electives, then make your own choice. Instead of choosing an elective that will "expedite things in graduate school," choose one that will help you survive undergraduate school. Trust your instincts. You may be smarter to pass up intermediate statistics and opt for art appreciation.

If you have difficulty persuading your advisors to let you take offbeat electives, remind them that art, music, and drama all have therapeutic applications. Call on their interests in the legal, ethical, economic, or political ramifications of health care. Convince them that public relations is currently receiving as much attention from the hospital hierarchy as patient care. Confess that you have international (or even interplanetary) aspirations for nursing.

If all else fails, produce this ad, which appeared in a big-city newspaper:

MEDICAL

RN
●●●●●

Unusually talented RN sought for intriguing position in long-term care setting. Requires flexibility, motivation, and strong nursing/teaching/social service skills. PR and marketing, sparkle, and a sense of humor a must. Call for interview appointment.

555-0000
EOE
●●●●●

Tell them that this is the job of your dreams and that you need this particular elective to improve your "sparkle" and "sense of humor." Sometimes an elective, just like this classified ad, brings much-needed comic relief. This ad shows that no elective should be deemed inappropriate.

Use the entire college catalog when you are searching for electives. Be brave. Boldly go where no nursing student has gone before. Explore! Enjoy!

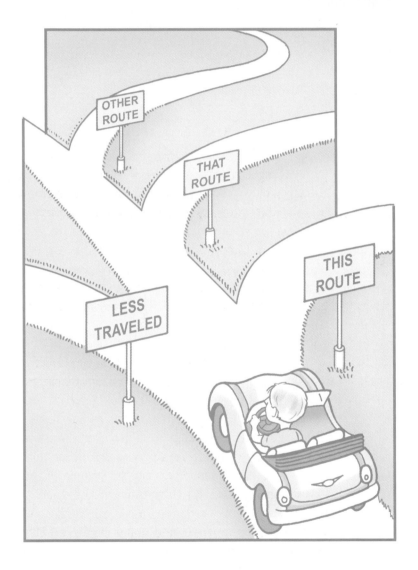

20

Alternative Routes

"Make it thy business to know thyself, which is the most difficult lesson in the world."
—Cervantes, *Don Quixote*

As you approach nursing, you may be surprised by the number of alternate routes available. Some nurses enjoy caring for children; others enjoy caring for the elderly. Some enjoy working in the emergency department; others enjoy working in intensive care, obstetrics, orthopedics, gastroenterology, or hospice nursing. If you thrive on delving into the subconscious, take the exit marked "Psychiatric Nursing." If you prefer the unconscious, take the "Operating Room" exit. You may veer off toward school nursing, occupational health nursing, or even private practice. The number of alternate routes will both delight and confuse you.

How do you know which route will be right for you? While you are in school, you will have several chances to sample alternate routes. Take full advantage of this opportunity. Push yourself to explore as many alternatives as possible.

When I taught at the University of Wisconsin–Madison, clinical experience in psychiatric nursing was an option, not a requirement. The students I had in this class were exceptional. Did they sign up because they thought they had an affinity for psychiatric nursing? No. Most of them were scared. They didn't *have* to come, and many confessed they didn't *want* to come, but they *chose* to come rather than miss a unique opportunity. All were glad they made the trip, even though only a few went on to become psychiatric nurses.

GET OUT AND PUSH

Instead of looking for an easy out or sliding along the path of least resistance, challenge yourself. Cultivate your adventurous streak. To increase your flexibility and tolerance, exercise. Stretch yourself to the limits. You don't have to abandon your goals or values, but you do need to test them. Examine their origins, their accuracy, and their usefulness.

When you hit the open road to nursing, the best thing you can bring along is an open mind. You will be caring for, and working with, people of every race, religion, creed, culture, sex, age, education, and income bracket. Tolerance and flexibility mean survival.

Nurses are supposed to be nonjudgmental—a noble concept that is impossible to attain. You will be judgmental. You will judge everyone on the basis of your standards, just as I will judge everyone on the basis of mine.

To keep judgmental attitudes from interfering with professional performance, you have to know yourself inside and out. Take a few moments to describe yourself by answering the following questions:

Age?
Sex?
Race?
Ethnic background?
Region of country?
Urban or rural?
Fat or thin?
Religion? How religious?
Political preference? How political?
Education?
Income level?
Pet peeves?
Favorite charities?
Energy level?
Optimistic or pessimistic?
Shy or bold?

Recreational pastimes or hobbies?

Dreams?

Fears?

Family commitments?

Et cetera?

The more answers you have in common with someone, the more comfortable you will be with that person. Unfortunately, you cannot choose your patients or classmates as you do your friends. You have to take what you get and then work at establishing a relationship. The operative word is *work*.

On the highway there is always a right side and a wrong side of the road. In nursing, as in life, the distinctions are not that clear-cut. Every day you will deal with sensitive people and emotionally charged issues. You need to be fully aware of your attitudes on abortion, euthanasia, pain control, venereal disease, suicide, disability, disfigurement, abuse, addiction, and the right to die—to name only a few.

When you find yourself holding views diametrically opposed to those of your patients, classmates, teachers, or co-workers, it is difficult to keep from being offended or from offending others. Knowing your feelings is crucial because attitudes guide actions.

In nursing you need to be able to tolerate a great deal of ambiguity. You have to learn to live with choices that are not yours to make.

Strive to recognize differences as differences. Steer clear of the impulse to label them as right or wrong. You can't live happily in nursing until you understand that your way is only one way. There will always be alternate routes.

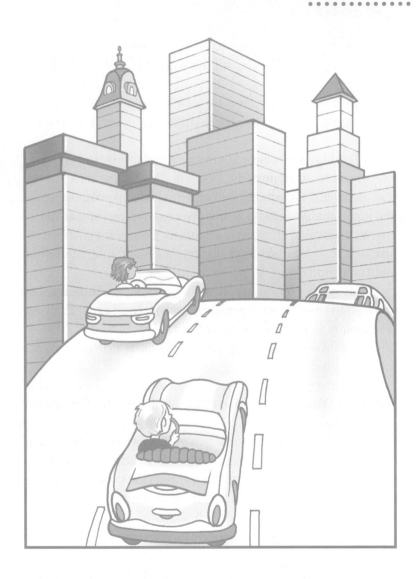

21

Business Routes

"…it has made me like working to see that writing is not a performance but a generosity."
—Brenda Ueland, *If You Want to Write*

When you are a student, your business is to deliver words on demand. Whether drafting a term paper, giving a report to the next shift, persuading an instructor to modify an assignment, writing a care plan, presenting an award, making a report to classmates, teaching a patient self-care, or addressing an international meeting, it all boils down to words.

When you need to get down to business, there are two routes you can follow. You can either deliver words in person, or you can deliver words on paper.

WORDS DELIVERED IN PERSON

When you have to deliver words in person, the first rule is to *know your audience.* Will there be one person or one hundred? Regular people or professionals? Male or female? Age? Education? Primary interests? Familiarity with the subject? The better you know your audience, the better your chances for a successful presentation.

Next, you have to know the *purpose* of your presentation. Are you supposed to stimulate interest, provide information, arouse to action, teach a skill, or entertain?

Consider how much time you have for your presentation. The amount of preparation time required for a good presentation is inversely proportional to the amount of time allotted. That means it takes more preparation time to give a good 10-minute talk than a good 60-minute talk. The less time you have to deliver your presentation, the more efficiently focused, tightly organized, and highly polished you have to be.

When you try to tell your audience "everything," they usually leave with nothing. Good presenters know how important it is to define and limit content.

To prioritize content, ask yourself, "If the audience could take away only *one* idea or piece of information, what should it be?" That becomes your first and foremost objective. What is the second most important idea for them to grasp? The third?

By prioritizing your content, you will know how much time and attention to devote to each section. And if you are allotted less time for your presentation than expected, you will know where to trim it without doing major damage.

The Construction

Taking the three vital objectives you have identified, draft a bare-bones outline. Do whatever reading, research, or interviewing is necessary to flesh it out.

Some students prefer to write out their speeches word for word. That is fine if you promise not to read it word for word. Never, ever read your speech. You will bore people to death. Never, ever memorize your speech. You will bore yourself to death.

After you've constructed a comprehensive outline or drafted your entire speech, grab a couple of index cards. Now: reduce your entire speech to a dozen key words or phrases.

The Rehearsal

Pick up your index cards and begin rehearsing. Play with alternate words and phrases. Then, when you stand before the audience, you will not suffer a loss for words or panic when you cannot remember the exact words.

Using a tape recorder during rehearsal is an excellent idea. Listening to yourself for the first time is often a shock. It may not sound like you to you, but that is the way you sound to others. Listen to your voice. Is it lively, well modulated, clear? Do you mumble, stammer, say "you know" 529 times? Check the pacing and your choice of words.

Resist the compulsion to fill every second with words such as "ah ... uh ... ahummm." Clearing your throat and coughing are usually nervous attempts to fill empty spaces. Actually, pauses and silences can have a powerful impact. With practice, you can learn to be comfortably quiet between thoughts.

Choose words that are positive. Make no apologies or excuses such as "I wish I had had more time to prepare" or "You probably know more about this subject than I do."

Do not talk down to your audience. Do not snow them with statistics or use half your time dropping names of experts. Steer clear of slang, jargon, and profanity.

Consciously curb nervous gestures such as twisting your hair, pulling your ears, blinking rapidly, giggling, playing with your notes, or jingling the change in your pocket.

Sometimes it helps to rehearse in front of a mirror. Then you can see yourself as others see you. This shock may be even greater than the one you get from listening to yourself on the tape recorder. But if you are serious about improving your speaking skills, you have to be willing to critique yourself. Poise will come with practice.

When you rehearse, go through your entire speech from start to finish. If you make a mistake or forget an important point, make a graceful recovery and keep going. You won't be able to start over from the beginning when you face a live audience.

You also need to time yourself during rehearsal. Inexperienced speakers invariably underestimate the amount of time it takes for delivery. With 2 minutes left, half of their content remains untouched. Remember, nothing makes an audience happier than a speaker who ends on time, unless it is a speaker who ends 5 minutes early.

Have a full dress rehearsal, especially if you plan to wear new clothes or shoes. Test drive your outfit so you know your shoes won't pinch, your skirt won't ride up, and you can reach the top of the chalkboard without splitting a seam. Choose something that is comfortable yet attractive and very professional looking.

Are you a little nervous about your presentation? Good. A bit of anxiety gets the adrenaline flowing and helps you do your best. An overdose of anxiety, however, can paralyze you.

The Countdown

There are several things you can do to keep anxiety under control. For example, visit the room where you will give your presentation. Check out the lighting, acoustics, exits, seating arrangements, the location of the nearest bathroom. Stand behind the lectern. Run through a few lines.

Decide where you will place any equipment or props. Practice using projectors or other mechanical devices.

If possible, mingle with the audience before your session begins. Introduce yourself, chat, eavesdrop. Learning a few names and faces can put things on a much friendlier basis.

If your throat is dry, take a sip of warm drink. Ironically, speakers are usually given a pitcher of ice water. A cold drink will contract throat muscles, but a warm one will relax them.

The Delivery

Take a deep breath. Concentrate on the audience, not on yourself. Make eye contact. Smile. Even if there are 300 people in the room, speak to one person at a time.

Engage your audience as much as possible. Draw them in and get them to nod in agreement with what you are saying.

Although you should never memorize your whole speech, there are two parts you should memorize: your opening line and your closing line. Knowing exactly how you will launch your speech will reduce anxiety. Knowing how you can bring your speech to an effective close lets you be more relaxed and responsive during your speech.

Be sensitive to your audience. Do not ignore their needs by hurrying through your speech. Watch them. If they seem confused, bored, overheated, or agitated, stop. Find out where the problem lies. You may need to open a window, close a door, take an unscheduled stretch break, give them an individual exercise, or allow them to make comments and ask questions.

If you are giving a presentation to your classmates and you have only one picture, chart, or model, do not pass it around the group while you are talking. It is too distracting. Either make a copy for everyone, convert the material to a slide, or offer to make it available after the session for anyone who wants a closer look.

Audiovisual aids make a presentation more interesting and enhance learning. Pictures are literally worth a thousand words. The audience will forget 90% of your words but will remember pictures and the ideas behind them.

Handouts can supplement information and reduce the need for note taking. If you are only going to discuss three aspects of cerebral palsy, you may want to make a list of "Twenty Facts About Cerebral Palsy" with a suggested reading list. Participants like to have something in hand that they can take home.

If someone asks a question and you don't know the answer, say, "I don't know the answer, but I will have it for you tomorrow." If you make a mistake, admit it. If someone challenges your information, be ready to cite sources. If he or she persists, offer to meet later to compare and contrast information. If someone is argumentative, don't become defensive. Say, "That is a very interesting point of view. I would like to continue this discussion when there is more time."

WORDS DELIVERED ON PAPER

When you have to deliver words on paper, you can follow many of the same principles that apply to delivering words in person. First, *know your audience.* Who is going to read this paper? Write for the reader.

Decide on the purpose of the paper. Are you attempting to inform, persuade, or entertain?

Consider the importance of the assignment. Is this a daily exercise or a paper that will constitute half of your grade?

The amount of time you invest should be proportional to the amount of benefit you expect to receive.

Next, choose a topic. Choosing is not as difficult as narrowing that topic down to a manageable size. Before you begin writing "Communicable Diseases Through the Ages" (a topic that would fill 10 volumes), talk to your instructor. You will probably end up writing something more like "Measles from 1910 to 1920." If you follow your instructor's advice and suggestions, success is almost guaranteed because your instructor is your reader.

Once you and your instructor have agreed on the topic, draft a brief outline. Then head for the library and the librarian. Librarians will direct you not only to current guides for nursing literature but also to computer services that can generate a list of all relevant articles published in the last few years. The fee is nominal and well worth it if your time is short.

Usually, your problem will be identifying quality articles. Occasionally, the problem is finding an adequate number of articles. A couple of years ago, I attended a meeting of the American Association for the Advancement of Science. One of the sessions, "The Oldest Old," was to focus on people over the age of 85 (the fastest growing segment of the population). When the sociologists who did the presentation went to the library to do research, they literally found nothing there. The subject was *too recent.*

Provided what you need is in print, your librarian can help you find it. Even if your school is small and your library is limited, the librarian can arrange interlibrary loans. Books and journals can be sent from major health science libraries.

A source I have found most helpful is *http://www.abebooks. com.* I wanted to write a children's book on Lillian Wald, a turn-of-the-20th-century New York nurse who developed the Visiting Nurse Service, created the occupation of school nurse, and built one of the very first public playgrounds. I found that only a dozen books had been written on Wald, and I bought all of them from Abe Books. I also bought the only two books she had written. Now, if you are a book collector, vintage books can be very expensive. But if you are a reader or researcher, you can get a perfectly usable book for a couple of bucks. The on-line bookseller saved me untold hours of time and made my research thoroughly enjoyable.

Before you spend much time reading any book or article, scan it. Titles are often misleading, and many that appear relevant are not.

As you read, watch for recurring themes, major issues, milestones, facts, and figures. Take notes on index cards. Keep track of questions that need answering.

Before you begin writing, refine your outline. Reorganize it and make it as comprehensive as possible. Decide which information carries the most weight. Prioritize objectives just as you did when you prepared your speech. What is the most important idea or piece of information? The second most important? The third?

Floor It

Let your fingers fly when you write the first draft. Pay no attention to spelling, punctuation, phrasing, or logic. Scribble thoughts as fast as they occur to you. Whether you write or type, leave wide margins and plenty of space between lines where you can rewrite or add information.

Set the paper aside. Sleep on it. The next morning, work it over. Edit, reorganize, expand. Strive for simple words and short sentences.

Write a second draft. If possible, let 2 or 3 days elapse, then work it over again. Reading your paper aloud is often helpful.

Sometimes when you work long and hard on a project, you cannot see its fatal flaws. Let a friend check your paper for readability, logic, and content. Ask for a double check on spelling and punctuation. If you have a word processing program with a spell checker, be sure to use it.

Just remember, even spell checkers have limitations. Here's a little ditty that made the rounds on the Internet:

ODE TO A SPELL CHECKER

I have a spelling checker,
It came with my P.C.;
It plainly marks four my revue,
Mistakes I cannot sea.

I've run this poem threw it,
I'm sure your please too no;
Its letter perfect in it's weigh,
My checker tolled me sew.

Formats for footnotes and bibliographies are varied. What is in vogue at one school will be inappropriate at another. Ask your instructor for guidelines. In an emergency, just follow the format in one of your recommended textbooks. As long as you are consistent in the way you handle references, you will not lose more than a couple of points.

When you print the final draft, use good-quality white paper (at least 20-pound, preferably with rag content). Make sure each page has a number and your name. Do a professional quality job on the title page and the cover. Neatness does count.

Finally, the only thing better than delivering your paper on time is delivering it ahead of schedule.

No matter what route you take after nursing school, skills as a speaker and writer will always help you.

"The difference between the right word and the almost right word is the difference between lightning and the lightning bug."
—Mark Twain

"No good deed goes unpunished."
—Clare Booth Luce

"The best thing about the future is that it comes only one day at a time."
—Abraham Lincoln

"The most pathetic person in the world is someone who has sight, but has no vision."
—Helen Keller

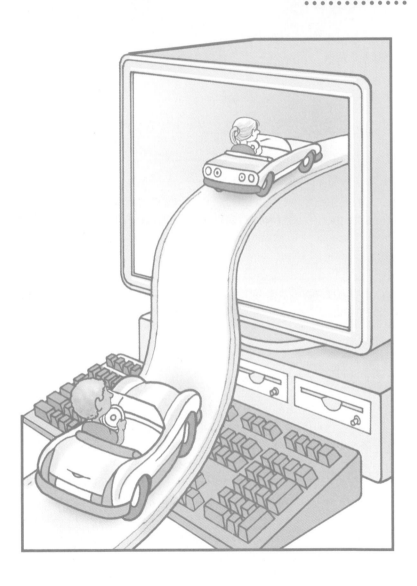

22

Hot-Wired

"The future is purchased by the present."
—Dr. Samuel Johnson

Whiplash. That's what you get when you try to keep up with changes on the Internet and the World Wide Web. Both offer unparalleled opportunities and unprecedented problems.

The book you are holding is revised every 5 years. Books on technology are being continuously revised. Before the ink dries, they are obsolete. One of my favorites is *The Internet for Dummies*, which has been revised eight times in 8 years. It does make your head spin. I hope this chapter will tickle your fancy and help you begin thinking about ways to use these technologies as a student and later as a nurse.

TICKET TO RIDE

You need four tickets to ride the Internet: a *computer;* a *modem,* which hooks your computer to phone or cable lines; an account with an *Internet provider;* and *software,* which allows you to navigate the Web.

Figuring out which hardware, software, or service to use is extremely frustrating because new options become available every 30 seconds. Just when you think you have finally acquired a state-of-the-art system, along comes one that is faster, more powerful, and worst of all—cheaper!

If you don't have your own equipment, you can get access to the Internet at schools, libraries, cyber cafes, or your workplace. However, many schools of nursing are now requiring students to have laptop computers and personal digital assistants (PDAs).

Classrooms are being equipped with wireless Internet access, and many instructors put their course materials online. You can e-mail your term papers and care plans and even take tests online. In the classroom, you can take class notes on your laptop. In the hospital, you can use your PDA to download the latest information on drugs, diseases, and treatments. You suddenly have the freedom and flexibility to work from home—or the beach! You can log on at noon or at midnight.

Being hot-wired lets you use e-mail (electronic mail). It's the best invention since the telephone, and it's on its way to making the post office almost obsolete. It is a fun, fast, inexpensive way to keep in touch with family and friends.

You can even keep in touch with people around the globe. A couple of years ago, I was invited to speak to a group of nurses in Japan. Two of my former classmates with nursing connections there went with me for a 10-day junket. In addition to sightseeing, we toured nursing schools, hospitals, and health care organizations in several cities. Today we can keep in touch with our newfound colleagues and friends via e-mail. It's quick, it's easy, and it's free! And you don't have to worry about time zones.

It's also a great way for classmates and teachers to keep in touch. Instead of driving to a study group, you can all log on and have a discussion online. If you have a question about an assignment or wonder where a test is being given, you can find out without playing telephone tag.

My daughter-in-law, Maria, locked her keys in the car on a Friday afternoon, the last day of the semester. She was frantic because she was going to miss a class in which she was required to turn in her final paper. While waiting for the locksmith, she e-mailed her paper to the professor, telling him what had happened. That way he would know that she hadn't skipped school because she hadn't done her homework. E-mail saved the day.

Whether you send messages by snail mail (the post office) or e-mail, you need an address. If you want to contact me, for example, you would type in melodie@pronurse.com.

Unfortunately, there are other companies that own similar domain names. Add a hyphen or a capital letter and you will be off to the wrong address.

Addresses on the Web usually end with a dot and three letters. For example:

.edu means an educational institution
.gov means a government agency
.mil means military
.com is a commercial site
.org means an organization

Many e-mail addresses are long and awkward to type. To save time use your "address book" feature. Type in the first couple of letters and the full address will pop up. There is also a "bookmark" feature that allows you to store your favorite websites. Just a click and you are there. It saves time and eliminates errors.

Communications on the Internet tend to be brief, breezy, informal, and often loaded with acronyms. For example, FAQ means frequently asked questions; BTW means by the way; FYI means for your information; and LOL means laughing out loud. There are certain rules of etiquette (called "netiquette"). For example, DO NOT TYPE YOUR MESSAGES IN CAPITAL LETTERS. It is considered shouting. It is rude. Besides, it is much more difficult to read. Be sure to use your dictionary or spell checker. It's never cool to look like a fool.

START YOUR ENGINES ... YOUR SEARCH ENGINES

To find what you are looking for on the Internet you need a search engine. There are several. I go to Google first, but other popular ones include Yahoo, Web Crawler, and Alta Vista.

The Internet can save you a lot of time and energy. You can check movie listings, compare auto prices, buy airline tickets, print out IRS tax forms, do a job search, check the weather around the world, find your best friend from kindergarten, tour an art museum in France, order office supplies, play the stock market, read an encyclopedia, or get a map with step-by-step directions to any address in any city.

The Internet can also help you waste an enormous amount of time. Easily distracted people can spend hours wandering around cyberspace. For some it is as addictive as drugs, alcohol, nicotine, or chocolate! (Remember the chapter on Detours?)

Spam, the Internet equivalent of junk mail, also eats up a lot of time. Unsolicited and unwanted messages pile up quickly. Offers for moneymaking schemes, Viagra, crude nudes and hot chicks, pseudo-charity scams, low-interest loans, tasteless jokes, chain letters, and hoaxes pour in each day. Although senders are legally required to include information about how to get off their mailing lists, many experts recommend that you just hit the delete button. They suggest that if you try to get off a list, it merely confirms that you exist and your address is passed on to hundreds of other spammers.

DON'T GIVE YOUR CAR KEYS TO THIEVES

Crooks and thieves seem to be the first to master new technology. So only use your credit cards on secure sites, never reveal passwords or personal identification numbers (PINs), and don't give out your Social Security number unless it is absolutely necessary.

Any product's greatest strength is also its greatest weakness. The Internet is rife with uses and abuses because it offers speed, open access, anonymity, and a lack of geographic boundaries.

Scams abound. The Federal Trade Commission (FTC) is finding it difficult to keep fraudulent health products off the Web. The agency advises consumers to be wary of any ad that includes phrases such as "scientific breakthrough," "secret ingredient," or "ancient remedy." Other indications that an ad might represent a scam include undocumented case histories or testimonials of "miracle cures" and claims that the government or the medical profession has conspired to keep this product from consumers. Another red flag is any product that is available from only one source. The FTC's home page has more advice on how to evaluate diet, health, and fitness products (*http://www.ftc.gov*).

SITE SEEING

If you are writing a term paper and need a specific fact, the Internet can deliver it in a fraction of a second. In the same length of time, the Internet can overwhelm you with more information than you could use in a lifetime.

Using the search engine, Google, I just typed in the word "cancer," and in 0.06 second I found there were 10,900,000 entries containing that word. When I typed in "breast cancer," I found 1,720,000 entries. For "breast cancer support groups," there were 324,000 entries; for "breast cancer support groups in Iowa," there were 10,400 entries; for "breast cancer support groups in Des Moines, Iowa," there were 1100 entries. As you can see, the more specific you are in the key words you choose, the less material you will have to sift through.

In 1993 there were only 130 websites. Today there are millions. Every school, organization, agency, business, and bozo has a website. I have one. If you don't, you will. I even know a 5-month-old baby who has his own website!

Thousands upon thousands of sites are dedicated to health. How do you know which sites provide accurate, reliable, ethical, and useful information? It is not easy.

First, consider the source. Check to see if the site is operated by a medical school, a teaching hospital, a government agency, a well-known consumer organization, an established support group, or a reputable professional. Be aware that drug companies, equipment manufacturers, and the like have a vested interest. They will tout their own products and publish "scientific work" only if it improves their bottom line.

The site should provide the names and credentials of its authors and researchers. You can do a quick search to see if these "world-class experts" have published anything in legitimate professional journals.

The site should tell you when it was last updated and should provide links to other compatible websites.

At *http://www.healthfinder.gov* you will find links to more than 1800 carefully selected health information websites. It also has feature articles on health topics. General health care information is arranged by age, race, and gender. The site offers a library plus information about hospitals, long-term care, health insurance, and prescriptions.

Here are a handful of sites you can check out. They are listed in alphabetical order and will provide you with a tiny sample of what is available to those who are hot-wired. I suggest that you and your fellow students make a game out of finding your favorite website of the month and sharing it with each other. Make your own personal directory. Keep it current. Websites tend to appear and disappear with little rhyme or reason.

Agency for Healthcare Research and Quality (AHRQ):
   http://www.ahcpr.gov
American Cancer Society: *http://www.cancer.org*
American Diabetes Association: *http://www.diabetes.org*
American Heart Association: *http://www.americanheart.*
   org
Food and Drug Administration: *http://www.fda.gov*
HealthAtoZ.com: *http://www.healthatoz.com*
Health On the Net Foundation: *http://www.hon.ch*
Mayo Clinic: *http://www.mayoclinic.org*
MEDLINE plus: *http://medlineplus.gov*
Medscape: *http://www.medscape.com*
National Institutes of Health (NIH): *http://www.nih.gov*
US Department of Health & Human Services: *http://www.*
   hhs.gov
US National Library of Medicine: *http://www.nlm.nih.gov*
WebMD: *http://www.webmd.com*
World Health Organization: *http://www.who.int*

It's wonderful to have access to the Library of Medicine, but you will not find the full text for many of the articles. You will primarily find abstracts—brief summaries—but that will be enough to tell you whether the article is worth tracking down. If you can't find the actual book or journal in your college library, you can get it through interlibrary loan.

Some online professional journals are free, but others have subscription fees just as printed journals do. The Internet lets you access articles from newspapers and popular magazines. Often, there is a small fee ($2.00 to $3.00) if you want to print it out. You can put it on your credit card.

Websites such as Medscape are free but require registration before you are given access. Medscape offers more than 100 medical journals, online continuing education, and daily medical news. Talk about a bargain!

IT BYTES!

Feeling invisible and anonymous, people visit places on the Internet they wouldn't dare go in real life. They think that if they just hit the delete button, no one will ever know where they went, what they did, or what they said. They think their actions will vanish without a trace into thin air. Wrong.

We've all seen the FBI confiscating the computers of suspected criminals, potential terrorists, sleazy businessmen, and mischievous teenage hackers on the evening news. The authorities can reconstruct all your activities.

If you visit bad neighborhoods, you better expect trouble. So don't visit pornography or hate group sites. Don't gamble, perpetrate hoaxes, participate in get-rich-quick schemes, pose nude, make racial slurs, or pass along obscene jokes.

Some students have purchased term papers online and submitted them as their own. Maybe I should say "former students." It is not just lazy; it is unethical. It may get you kicked out of college or cost you your scholarship.

A University of Virginia physics professor, Louis A. Bloomfield, wrote a software program that compared student papers. He was able to identify 122 students who had copied paragraphs or entire papers from those of previous students and submitted them as their own. They were high-tech cheaters who were caught with high-tech methods. Poetic justice.

TELEPHONE, TELEVISION … TELEHEALTH???

Telehealth is an odd word with great possibilities. Basically, it is the use of telecommunications networks and equipment (computer, phone, fax, radio, cable, and video) to transfer health information and provide health care.

Think of it as remote-control care. There are times when it is impossible or not feasible for professionals and patients to meet face to face. Consider mountain climbers, astronauts, soldiers on the battlefield, victims of natural disasters, or the elderly in an isolated rural area.

While the word may not be familiar to you, we've been dabbling in telehealth for more than 50 years. That's when the first video conferencing enabled health care professionals to share information and provide education simultaneously to groups around town or around the world. Thirty years ago, nurses and emergency medical technicians began transmitting vital patient information from accident scenes to physicians in the hospital. Doctors were able to make long-distance diagnoses and prescribe life-saving treatment that could begin immediately.

Today, interest in telehealth is skyrocketing because of exciting developments, including widespread access, affordability, and the enhanced capabilities of new computers and networks.

We already have telemedicine and telenursing, but maybe we should coin a new word, *telepatient*, because patients are also online. They come to their doctors' appointments with printouts of information about the disease, fatality rates, standard medications, and experimental treatments. Many are not only informed, they are misinformed. Part of your professional responsibility will be helping them differentiate rumors from facts and doctors from quacks. (You may want to refer them to *http://www.quackwatch.com*.)

Telepatients may medicate themselves with drugs purchased online. Every conceivable drug is offered at bargain prices, and no pesky prescription is needed. Whether the drugs are real or fake, pure or contaminated is anybody's guess. This is one of the Internet's dangers.

On a more positive note, telepatients have spontaneously formed support groups for every imaginable problem. Medical experts can talk the talk, but patients want first-hand information from experienced fellow sufferers and their families. They want to hear from those who have actually lived with their disease or disability. Support group members lend sympathetic ears. They dispense no-nonsense advice and offer prayers. They share suggestions and make recommendations. They offer down-to-earth problem-solving tips. When a message is sent out, even in the middle of the night, someone in the group will respond. It's always daylight somewhere in the world, and support groups span the globe! Patients say the biggest comfort is knowing that they are not alone and not crazy.

BOLDLY GO

Participants in telehealth must also solve some unprecedented problems. Even if everyone is online, we all have different hardware and software. Some systems are incompatible and cannot communicate with one another. Billing patients for e-mail visits and video consultations must be worked out. It takes time, money, and personnel to digitize data. Doctors and nurses have been slow to adapt to and adopt these new technologies. Professional licenses are issued by the state. With telehealth you will need a national license, an international license, or perhaps an intergalactic license!

Finally, every professional group is going to have to develop professional standards and codes of conduct as we boldly go where no health care system has gone before.

THE AMERICAN NURSES ASSOCIATION'S CORE PRINCIPLES ON TELEHEALTH

1. The basic standards of professional conduct governing each health care profession are not altered by the use of telehealth technologies to deliver health care, conduct research, or provide education. Developed

by each profession, these standards focus in part on the practitioner's responsibility to provide ethical and high-quality care.

2. A health care system or health care practitioner cannot use telehealth as a vehicle for providing services that are not otherwise legally or professionally authorized.

3. Services provided via telehealth must adhere to basic assurances of quality and professional health care in accordance with each health care discipline's clinical standards. Each health care discipline must examine how telehealth affects or changes its patterns of care delivery and what modifications to existing clinical standards may be required.

4. The use of telehealth technologies does not require additional licensure.

5. Each health care profession is responsible for developing its own processes for ensuring competencies in the delivery of health care through the use of telehealth technologies.

6. Practice guidelines and clinical guidelines in the area of telehealth should be developed based on empirical evidence, when available, and on professional consensus among all involved health care disciplines. The development of these guidelines may include collaboration with government agencies.

7. The integrity and therapeutic value of the client–health care practitioner relationship should be maintained and not diminished by the use of telehealth technology.

8. Confidentiality of client visits, client health records, and the integrity of information in a health care information system are essential.

9. Documentation requirements for telehealth services must be developed that ensure documentation of each client encounter with recommendations and treatments, communication with other health care

providers as appropriate, and adequate protections for client confidentiality.

10. All clients directly involved in a telehealth encounter must be informed about the process, the attendant risks and benefits, and their rights and responsibilities. Clients must provide adequate informed consent.

11. The safety of clients and practitioners must be ensured. Safe hardware and software, combined with demonstrated user competency, are essential components of safe telehealth practice.

12. A systematic and comprehensive research agenda must be developed and supported by government agencies and health care professions for the ongoing assessment of telehealth services.

Reprinted with permission from the American Nurses Association. *Core Principles on Telehealth.* Washington, DC: American Nurses Publishing, American Nurses Foundation/American Nurses Association, 1999.

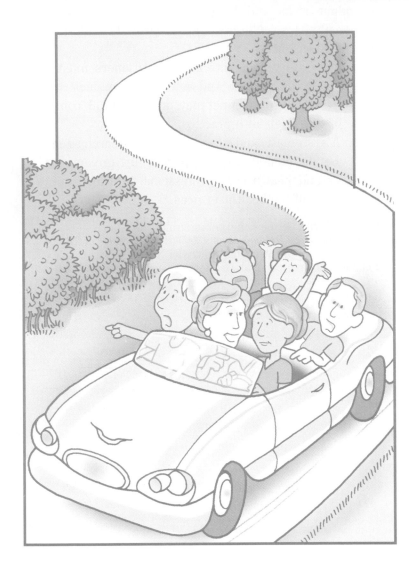

23

In the Driver's Seat

"Experience is the name everyone gives to his mistakes."
—Oscar Wilde

A few feet off the interstate, the exit split into northbound and southbound lanes. The driver ahead of me was obviously unsure which lane was the "right" lane. Before he could make up his mind, he impaled his car on the lane divider.

If he had it to do over again, I am sure he would agree that even the "wrong" decision would have been better than no decision. He may have had to drive a little out of his way, but he would have arrived in one piece.

In a moving vehicle, decision time is limited. To be a good driver, you need a ready mind and a steady hand. You need to size up situations quickly, make decisions, and take action.

The same is true of nursing.

When you are in the driver's seat, you take full responsibility for your actions. When you make an error, you must take the consequences. Even if some backseat driver gave you a bum steer, the citation will be issued to you.

The same is true of nursing.

Professionally speaking, when you are in the driver's seat, you take full responsibility for your actions. When you make an error, and you will, do not waste time making excuses. Face up to your responsibility. Learn from the experience. Then drive on.

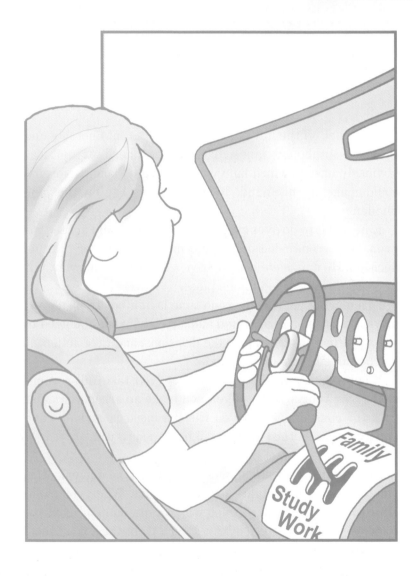

24

Shifting Gears

"Life does not cease to be funny when people die any more than it ceases to be serious when people laugh."
—George Bernard Shaw

Going back to school after several years' absence can be a real jolt to the system. The song goes, "I will never pass this way again," and yet here you are back in school at 25, 30, 40, or 50 years of age.

Consider what happened to my sister. She is a business whiz. When a golden opportunity appeared, she did not see the need to finish college. She signed on with a rapidly expanding company and, through a combination of sheer talent and incredibly hard work, rose to a vice president's position. She was on the fast track and confident that she had it made. Until her company merged. She found herself out on the street with several other top-level managers.

She quickly discovered that it was impossible to get a comparable position without proper academic credentials. Oh, there were jobs available but not the career opportunities she wanted. For example, one representative told her his company would not even interview her for a *secretarial* position without a bachelor's degree. She soon found herself back in school—a little older, a little wiser.

People who find themselves back in school at midlife are called "mature" students. Whether this is a first career venture, a move to enhance career options, or a complete career change makes little difference. In addition to the academic challenge, there are a multitude of other stressors.

VINTAGE VEHICLE

Mature students don't worry about a date for homecoming. They worry about coming home and finding that the babysitter has quit. The cupboard is bare, the toilet is overflowing, the dog is in heat, and the mortgage is due. Meeting obligations means continually making tough choices and uncomfortable compromises.

Many mature students have to commute. They can't relocate their families, so they "dislocate" themselves.

"I was a full-time student at the university with a husband 200 miles away who claimed he couldn't cook for himself. I drove 200 miles on Friday to cook, clean, be the ideal wife on Saturday and Sunday. I drove back Sunday evening and spent the whole night studying for the week. Both grades and marriage came out intact, but I was physically and mentally exhausted."

A long drive to and from school can be a grueling experience. Here is how one student came to enjoy her roadwork.

"I spend 12 hours away from home at least 5 days a week. My 'spare time' is spent driving 2 hours each day to and from school. At first I resented the drive. Now I love it. I can sing all four parts to the choir songs. I love to listen to the news and the games. I recognize certain cars and trucks; we honk and wave. I share a common bond with their drivers. Life has so many perks if you just look for them. My 2 hours behind the wheel have become a gift instead of a burden."

Maintaining a positive attitude and accepting the drive as part of the price of higher education will make the road seem shorter. Don't waste time and energy resenting reality. Go with it.

The road to nursing always goes uphill. If you want to make it to the top, you have to shift to a lower gear and lighten your load as much as possible. This is especially true for married students and those with children, regardless of age.

Married men have an advantage. They have wives. Married women have a disadvantage. They *are* wives.

Being a wife-mother-student means going into overdrive. After spending all day in class and clinical, you race home (driven by guilt), toss in a load of laundry, start dinner, vacuum the living room, balance the checkbook, check the kids' homework, walk the dog, and listen to an instant replay of your husband's day at work. When you finally get everyone bedded down for the night, you tiptoe to the kitchen table, spread out your books, and study until past midnight. The next morning you wake up tired and already behind schedule.

Many women fail to make the grade in nursing school because they refuse to lighten their loads. They vow that nothing will change. They try valiantly to do everything just as before, but they fall farther and farther behind. Women drive themselves too hard.

They've Found Something That Can Do the Work of Ten Men ...

Participants at a Midwestern nursing management conference included approximately 100 women and *only one man*. All held demanding jobs in middle and upper management. The afternoon session dealt with the Superwoman complex— the compulsion to do everything perfectly, from cooking to cleaning to parenting to advancing a career.

The man, who was still a bachelor, was amazed at what he heard. He didn't see how the women could manage to do everything at work and everything at home. It had never occurred to him that he should do his own housework. As soon as he was employed, he had hired someone to come in twice a week.

It doesn't occur to men to do their own housework. It doesn't occur to women *not* to do their own housework. Time to shift!

After that conference, many of those nurse-managers probably hired housekeeping help. As a student you may not be able to afford help, yet you cannot afford to be without it. If you can't hire it, you have to commandeer it.

Just as it never occurred to the male manager to do his own housework, it will probably never occur to your husband to do *his* own housework. Studies show that husbands of working wives do no more household chores than husbands of nonworking wives. Chances are that this holds true for children, too. If you want your family's help around the house, you will have to be the one who says so.

Make lists of essential household chores and let family members choose which ones they prefer to do. Divide the ones nobody wants and assign them on a rotating basis. Have some chores available for extra credit. These pay bonuses over allowances.

Dancing in the Dust

An Iowa student found that she could get the whole family to pitch in for 1 hour every Saturday morning. They turned on rock-and-roll music, and all six of them danced through the house doing their assigned chores.

If dancing house cleaners don't measure up to your exacting standards, relax your standards. In fact, if you are going to survive nursing school, you have to relax, period.

Family members can feel threatened as your friends, interests, lifestyle, and priorities shift. There may be some anger, fear, jealousy, and resentment. There can also be new joy, pride, fun, and adventure.

Who *Is* This Person?

Nursing absorbs so much time and attention that one man complained that he had to make an appointment just to see his wife. A lot of the romance and spontaneity seemed to have gone out of their relationship. Their solution? They stopped thinking of their times together as "appointments" and began thinking of them as "dates." It revitalized their marriage.

The spouse always plays a critical role in the student's success or failure.

"As a diploma nurse the push is to get a degree and move on to a master's. When I was married with three children and a full-time job, I started back to school. My husband was very nonsupportive.

'That is more time away from me and the children.' I felt guilty about that too, but I was also angry. I had supported my husband through his last year of college and 4 years of postgraduate work. I went ahead with school but eventually dropped out. I guess the guilt and nonsupport weakened me. I'm now divorced with a full-time job, three children, less money, and going to school because my job requires a bachelor's."

How supportive is your spouse?

NO SUPPORT   **FULL SUPPORT**

☐ ☐

Be honest. Support is not just talk: it's ACTION! As a student prepared to head for the library one evening, her husband groaned, "Do I have to babysit again?" She snapped back, "No, you don't have to babysit. The only children here tonight will be yours!"

When long-established patterns are disrupted, when standard operating procedures are violated, tensions mount and tempers flare. In many ways the whole family goes back to school. Everyone is learning, adjusting, and adapting.

As you return to school, it's nice to have the support of friends and family. Not every student is that fortunate.

"Upon deciding I wanted a career—not just a job—I pledged to give it my all. My parents and relatives did not understand. My husband has ALWAYS been supportive, but comments from those 'outside' our lives really hurt. They would say things like 'You sure are neglecting your husband' or "It's too bad you can't spend more time together' or 'YOU can do that; YOU don't have children.' I decided to set my own goals and do what was needed to attain them. I have been successful. Whether other people support me or not, I made the decision that this is MY life and I'm doing these things for ME!!!"

How important is it for you to have the approval of family and friends? Can you stand alone? Can you say with this student, "This is MY life and I'm doing these things for ME!!!"? If you can, your chances of success are much greater.

Kiddie Care

The more support you have from your children, the better your chances of surviving nursing school. Let them know that things will be different. Help your family make the shift.

Involve your children as soon as possible and as much as possible. Talk to them about your school. Take them to the library, your classroom, the nursing skills laboratory, and the hospital. Children are much more comfortable when they can visualize where their parents are.

Make your children NURSE KITS. Toss in syringes, tongue blades, bandages, finger cots—whatever you can scrounge. Buy them a stethoscope of their own.

One family had "study hall" around the dining room table from 7:00 to 8:30 PM. Another family had each member go to a separate room and close the door for a "quiet hour."

To survive you need a private place where you can study. Privacy is something mothers are not supposed to need. Moms are supposed to be accessible 24 hours a day, 7 days a week, 365 days a year. Shift!

Go to your room. Close your door for 1 hour. Let an older child or your spouse handle problems and answer questions. When you emerge from study time, be ready to give your full, undivided attention to the family. If they know you will be really available at a certain time, they will permit you a study hour.

Even though you can't do everything together, you can do the important things together. What are the most important things? Ask your child. "What's one thing you would like us to do together today?" It may be having a special story read, hosting a tea party in the tree house, shopping for new tennis shoes, going to the zoo, working on a school project, or playing Monopoly. Let your children help plan special evenings, weekend outings, or vacation events.

Recognize that although you can do *anything*, you cannot do *everything*. You have to make choices.

For example, while driving across the country one summer, we decided to take a 200-mile detour and spend one day in a city where we had lived for several years. How could we see everyone in just 24 hours? We couldn't. So each of us chose the one person we most wanted to see. When we entered the city limits, we phoned the four people and made arrangements to see them. Then we drove to our old neighborhood and fit in other people and activities as we could. We left bright and early the next morning, feeling very satisfied and happy that we had made the detour.

WOMEN DRIVERS

One of the most popular workshops I teach is designed for women who are trying to do it all, have it all, and be it all. I call it "Walk-On-Water Women" (WOW for short). I ask participants to describe a situation in which two or more of their roles are in conflict. Many of the examples involve women who are back in school and trying to be good wives, good mothers, good daughters, good neighbors, good employees, and good students SIMULTANEOUSLY! It is exhausting.

In her fascinating book, *Sequencing*, Arlene Rossen Cardozo talks about women who have chosen to do it all, but not simultaneously. These women have had the foresight or the fortitude or the good fortune to have completed their education, established themselves firmly in careers, and then chosen to experience full-time mothering. I would call this sequencing with a capital "S." And I personally know of only one woman who has managed to pull this off.

For the rest of us—the frantic, the frazzled—who are trying to do it all simultaneously, I would like to recommend sequencing with a small "s." It begins with acknowledging that you cannot be in two places at once.

"Sometimes I feel torn—I'm working and in school, and on weekends I need to clean house, do laundry, scrub floors, cut grass, etc., etc., etc. My husband wants to do something fun for the weekend. I feel the need to spend time with him and the family, but then I have twice as much work to do when I return home—tired kids, dirty laundry, messy house. Most of the time I give in and then pay the price later for the fun. But again, sometimes I don't enjoy myself much because I know what's waiting for me when I get home—AND return to work and school THE NEXT DAY! Sometimes I resent my husband for not being able to see the work that needs to be done at home."

Here is another student with the same conflict but a much healthier way of handling it:

"When do I feel stressed? When behind in classes and housework and needing to do a million things at home! Like last Saturday when hubby and kids wanted to go to the cottage for a day but I didn't—I wanted to get caught up. This caused a conflict between my needs and theirs. After a 'discussion' the family went without me. I got everything done and felt good about the day. They came home having had a great day, and we wondered why we had argued."

In nursing school your social life will be sharply curtailed. With little time for family, you will have almost no time for friends. Say goodbye to dinner parties and hello to potlucks. You can also invite friends over just for dessert, or you can have a taco party to which everyone brings his or her favorite ingredient. True friends don't come for the food; they come for the fun of being together, and true friends won't mind if your house was cleaned by six rock-and-roll dancers.

Socialize with your classmates and their families. Families can compare notes, swap stories, sympathize with each other, and help solve problems.

Always have contingency plans. If the babysitter falls through, who is the backup person? If one of the children is sick, who will stay home? If the car breaks down, what alternate transportation is available? Contingency plans include a spare house key hidden in the flower pot, a spare lasagna in the freezer, a spare $20 bill under the mattress, and a spare uniform in the closet. Then you can shift at a moment's notice.

PROFESSIONAL DRIVERS

Whether male or female, young or old, you have to be able to shift gears when you enter the hospital. You must switch to your professional gear. For instance, people two or three times your age will be asking *you* for advice. They will tell you things they wouldn't tell their best friend, their spouse, or their clergy. You must respect these confidences, always protecting your patients' privacy and dignity.

With some practice, shifting from the personal to the professional mode becomes almost automatic. There are times, however, when that shift must be a conscious, deliberate decision.

For example, one nurse had some nagging personal problems that began interfering with her ability to concentrate at work. One day she noticed a large laundry basket parked outside the operating room area. As she passed by, she decided to dump her personal problems mentally into that basket. At the end of her shift, she mentally picked up her personal problems. Turning her personal life off during working hours made her happier and more productive. After work, even though she "picked up" her problems again, she felt better able to carry them. She approached her personal life with a new freshness and was able to resolve her problems in a short time.

MAKING THE GRADE

Mature students are often more uptight about grades than their younger counterparts. They feel driven to excel. Perhaps it is one way to justify all the time, energy, and money being diverted into school. Perhaps mature students want to set a good example for their own children. Whatever their motivation, they don't want to be good students—they want to be great.

Grades can become more important than learning. I know it's true. I've been there. I have spent a major portion of my life as a student. I feel like the fellow who quipped, "I've been in school so long I know things that just ain't so."

Like other overachievers, I have my own private grading system. If I get an A, I'm not always sure I earned it. I know I could have done more, learned more. If I get a B, I'm upset because Suzie-Q got an A, and I know I'm just as smart and worked just as hard as she did. If I get a C, I'm destroyed. For a highly competitive person like me, that's an automatic failure.

When I approached graduate school, I wanted things to be different. First of all, I wanted to combine psychiatric and pediatric nursing, but no such program existed. I devised one of my own. I took electives, did extra reading, and arranged my clinical assignments to reflect my private agenda. While conforming on the surface, below the surface I was busily doing my own thing.

I knew that if I let my grades influence me, I would neglect my own priorities. So I chose not to know my grades. To receive your grades at the University of Washington, you had to turn in a set of stamped, self-addressed envelopes. I didn't turn in any envelopes. I did not see my grades the entire time I was in graduate school. I figured if I were in academic trouble, someone would tap me on the shoulder and tell me to shape up. If I were doing OK, then it was just that—OK! The pursuit of perfection wouldn't sidetrack me.

During my fourth quarter I discovered what a liberating experience it had been. Evidently, one faculty member was a notoriously unfair grader. My fellow students were up in arms, ready to get tar and feathers. I just smiled to myself. I didn't know my grade. It honestly didn't matter to me. I had learned what I wanted to learn and had already moved on to other things.

Sometimes the only way to get where YOU really want to go is to shift gears and "brake" with old habits and traditions. Do whatever it takes to make sure learning is more important than grading.

BUYING AMERICAN OR JAPANESE?

When educational psychologists gave an unsolvable math problem to groups of Japanese and American children, they uncovered one key as to why our academic achievement is so much lower. The American kids struggled briefly and then gave up. The Japanese kids kept working, apparently believing that if you persist you can solve any problem.

Hard work is the key to success. Yet many Americans believe the key to success is inborn talent. Either you have it or you don't. Educational psychologists say our obsession with natural talent and innate ability has produced kids who give up easily. In fact, many Americans believe people who work hard in school must lack ability.

If you believe people are born smart, chances are you're a quitter. If you believe people are made smart, you'll knuckle down, persevere, and succeed! You'll know what Thomas Edison knew—that genius is 1% inspiration and 99% perspiration.

Being able to shift gears quickly is essential if you are to survive nursing school. From now on, you will have to shift more; "shiftless" students won't make it.

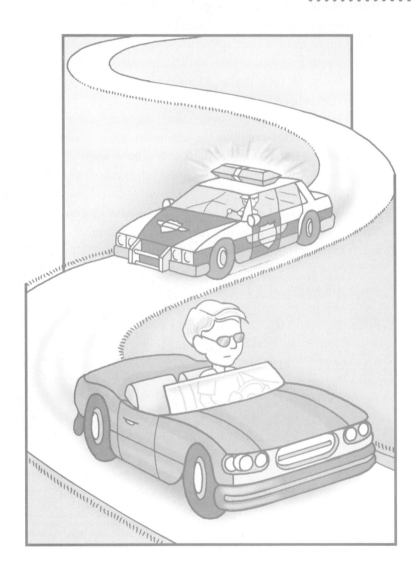

25

Moving Violations

"Well, Mrs. Upjohn, I guess I know my business. Of course, that's just a guess on my part."
—Groucho Marx, *A Day at the Races*

The summer before I went to nursing school, I worked a couple of months as a nurses' aid. I received no training or orientation. I was dumped directly on a busy floor during the evening shift. The nurse in charge would teach me the ropes as she had time.

I ran errands, fetched water, delivered dinner trays, and then was assigned to help patients get ready for bed, which included giving backrubs. The charge nurse told me to use lotion and powder.

My first "victim" was Maxine, a patient quite debilitated with multiple sclerosis. I smeared lotion all over her broad back and then liberally sprinkled powder on top. The two ingredients combined to form a lumpy paste. The more I rubbed, the worse it got.

Maxine shrieked, "Good grief, girl, what do you think you're doing!?" I replied, "Making pie crust." She burst into laughter.

I explained it was my first night, and I really had no idea of what I was doing. Immediately, she became my teacher. I learned a lot of basics from Maxine, including how tough it is to be a patient. She wrote to me while I was a nursing student, and, whenever I got home, I went to see her. She died shortly after I graduated.

Fortunately, you won't be tossed into the hospital in such a casual way. Before you hit the road, you will receive a lot of instruction.

Most of us had a driver's education course, and before we were allowed on the road, we spent hours reading, studying, and testing. There were films, demonstrations, discussions, and simulators to approximate driving conditions so that we could rehearse responses to all sorts of situations. When we passed the first part of the course, we were allowed to get behind the wheel of a specially equipped car. At our side sat an instructor using a dual-control system to keep us from making any dangerous errors. After we passed both written and driving exams, our licenses were granted. For the first time we were allowed to drive solo.

Nursing education follows much the same pattern. Before you are allowed to touch a patient, you spend hours reading, studying, testing, and rehearsing all sorts of technical procedures. If you are successful in the nursing skills laboratory, an instructor will accompany you to the patient for a real test of your ability. The instructor is there to protect you and your patient from any serious error. If you pass the patient test, you are allowed to do the procedure solo.

Being able to pass the "patient test" is crucial. If you fail the clinical portion of the course, you fail the course. There is no grade averaging here. Even straight-A students who fail clinical are out. The course must be repeated.

Mastering the skills and procedures of nursing practice is essential. To survive in nursing you must be able to use your hands as well as your head.

Of the students who botch the clinical component, only one in a thousand is a complete klutz. The others are usually ill-prepared or experience acute anxiety attacks that interfere with their performance.

To be well prepared you need to make the most of your time in the nursing skills lab. While waiting for your turn, you can learn a lot from your classmates. Keep alert. Watch every movement. Listen to the instructor's comments and the responses of your classmates. Envision yourself in your classmate's place. Feel the equipment in your hand. Anticipate each step. Recite the rationale to yourself. Concentrate.

USING YOUR HEAD

Sports experiments have repeatedly confirmed the value of "synthetic" experience. For example, in a classic study, students were divided into three groups and then tested on their ability to shoot free throws. For almost 3 weeks after the initial testing, group 1 practiced shooting free throws, group 2 did nothing related to basketball, and group 3 spent 20 minutes every day *imagining* they were shooting free throws. At the final test, group 2 showed no improvement, but groups 1 and 3 improved 24% and 23%, respectively. Studies like this one indicate that the human nervous system cannot distinguish between an actual experience and a vividly imagined one.

Picture Perfect

If you picture yourself failing, you double your chances of failure. If you picture yourself succeeding, you double your chances of success. So picture yourself doing the procedure and doing it perfectly, with precision and finesse. Mentally rehearse.

To control your anxiety, take slow, deep breaths. Focus on the patient and his or her needs. Recognize that sweaty palms, cold feet, butterflies in the stomach, and lightheadedness are normal symptoms of anxiety. Once the procedure is complete, they will disappear.

Be assured that you will never be permitted to perform a procedure on a patient that you haven't perfected in the skills lab. Remember, the instructor will be right by your side to coach you and to keep you from doing harm.

The first time you perform any procedure is nerve-racking at best. Some students keep trying to postpone the inevitable. They keep their heads down and stand at the back of the group, hoping they won't be chosen. Although it is possible to get through nursing school with minimum experience, it is not possible to get through with *no* experience.

Every time you postpone doing a procedure, anxiety builds until it reaches panic proportions. Confidence is the only cure, and confidence comes from competence. Competence comes from experience, and experience often comes the hard way. So keep your head up, stand at the front of the group, and volunteer.

I asked nurses what they would suggest students do to help take the terror out of clinical experience. Here is what they said:

"Remember that you are a student and there to learn. So ask questions and don't be afraid of not being perfect."

"Take a deep breath and say, I'm OK! I can do it!"

"Believe in yourself. Don't sweat the small stuff!!!"

"Don't ever be afraid to ask how to do something or admit you don't know an answer. We've all been in your shoes."

"We were all students once—remind us of what it's like. Ask for help and guidance."

"Don't tell the patient this is your first time. It isn't. You've practiced this over and over in the classroom."

"Just put yourself in the patient's place and think about how you would like to be treated."

"Relax. Be calm. The patient is a person just like you."

"Determine what will REALISTICALLY happen if you goof or screw up. The patient won't die and neither will you."

"Blow the situation so out of proportion that you'll laugh. Picture yourself and the patient as cartoon characters."

"Remember every nurse from the director of nursing on down had to take this first step."

"Don't let your instructor intimidate you. Remember, she was once a terrified student like you."

"Actually, your instructor wants you to pass/excel even more than you do. Think about it! If you don't look good, she doesn't look good. She's cheering for you."

"Pray."

"The first time is always terrifying. Go on—do it! The second time it feels better and works better."

"Realize anyone can make a mistake. There is no such thing as a bad experience. Always look for the positive. What have I learned from this?"

"Don't be afraid or embarrassed to try. Even if you blunder, remember doing is learning. It leads to confidence. Grab every experience you can!"

To get adequate experience, you may not only need to volunteer, you may have to fight to volunteer. Time in the clinical area is limited, and the procedures available are at a premium. You may get only one opportunity to perform a certain procedure. Once is not enough to build confidence or competence. To get more than minimum experience, make sure the staff knows which procedures you need to practice and which ones you are allowed to do solo. Make sure they know you are ready, willing, and able.

In driving and in nursing, the most serious infractions are moving violations. To keep from being labeled "unsafe at any speed," practice, practice, practice.

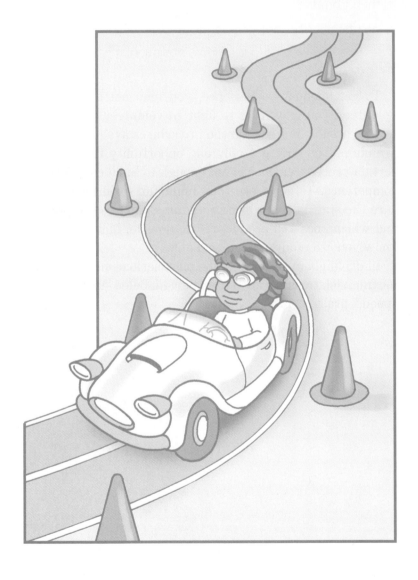

26

Defensive Driving

"In nature, there are neither rewards nor punishments; there are consequences."
—Robert Green Ingersoll

When you drive defensively, you protect yourself by watching out for the other guy. In many ways, watching out for the other guy is the very essence of nursing. Caring for and about others is our business. We have traditionally been more concerned about the rights of others than about our own rights.

Delineating "the other guy's" rights has become a national pastime. Every conceivable group has a "bill of rights." Patients have several champions. For example, here is the American Hospital Association's version of a patient's bill of rights. It was first adopted in 1973 and revised in 1992 and 2003.

THE PATIENT CARE PARTNERSHIP: UNDERSTANDING EXPECTATIONS, RIGHTS, AND RESPONSIBILITIES

When you need hospital care, your doctor and the nurses and other professionals at our hospital are committed to working with you and your family to meet your health care needs. Our dedicated doctors and staff serve the community in all its ethnic, religious, and economic diversity. Our goal is for you and your family to have the same care and attention we would want for our families and ourselves.

The sections explain some of the basics about how you can expect to be treated during your hospital stay. They also cover what we will need from you to care for you better. If you have questions at any time, please ask them. Unasked or unanswered questions can add to the stress of being in the hospital. Your comfort and confidence in your care are very important to us.

What to Expect During Your Hospital Stay

High-quality hospital care. Our first priority is to provide you the care you need, when you need it, with skill, compassion, and respect. Tell your caregivers if you have concerns about your care or if you have pain. You have the right to know the identity of doctors, nurses, and others involved in your care, and you have the right to know when they are students, residents, or other trainees.

A clean and safe environment. Our hospital works hard to keep you safe. We use special policies and procedures to avoid mistakes in your care and keep you free from abuse or neglect. If anything unexpected and significant happens during your hospital stay, you will be told what happened, and any resulting changes in your care will be discussed with you.

Involvement in your care. You and your doctor often make decisions about your care before you go to the hospital. Other times, especially in emergencies, those decisions are made during your hospital stay. When decision-making takes place, it should include:

Discussing your medical condition and information about medically appropriate treatment choices. To make informed decisions with your doctor, you need to understand:

- The benefits and risks of each treatment.
- Whether your treatment is experimental or part of a research study.

- What you can reasonably expect from your treatment and any long term effects it might have on your quality of life.
- What you and your family will need to do after you leave the hospital.
- The financial consequences of using uncovered services or out-of-network providers.

Please tell your caregivers if you need more information about treatment choices.

Discussing your treatment plan. When you enter the hospital, you sign a general consent to treatment. In some cases, such as surgery or experimental treatment, you may be asked to confirm in writing that you understand what is planned and agree to it. This process protects your right to consent to or refuse a treatment. Your doctor will explain the medical consequences of refusing recommended treatment. It also protects your right to decide if you want to participate in a research study.

Getting information from you. Your caregivers need complete and correct information about your health and coverage so that they can make good decisions about your care. That includes:

- Past illnesses, surgeries or hospital stays.
- Past allergic reactions.
- Any medicines or dietary supplements (such as vitamins and herbs) that you are taking.
- Any network or admission requirements under your health plan.

Understanding your health care goals and values. You may have health care goals and values or spiritual beliefs that are important to your well-being. They will be taken into account as much as possible throughout your hospital stay. Make sure your doctor, your family, and your care team know your wishes.

Understanding who should make decisions when you cannot. If you have signed a health care power of attor-

ney stating who should speak for you if you become
unable to make health care decisions for yourself, or
a "living will" or "advance directive" that states your
wishes about end-of-life care, give copies to your doctor,
your family, and your care team. If you or your family
need help making difficult decisions, counselors,
chaplains, and others are available to help.

Protection of your privacy. We respect the confidentiality of your relationship with your doctor and other
caregivers, and the sensitive information about your
health and health care that are part of that relationship.
State and federal laws and hospital operating policies
protect the privacy of your medical information. You
will receive a Notice of Privacy Practices that describes
the ways that we use, disclose, and safeguard patient
information and that explains how you can obtain a copy
of information from our records about your care.

Preparing you and your family for when you leave the
hospital. Your doctor works with hospital staff and
professionals in your community. You and your family
also play an important role in your care. The success of
your treatment often depends on your efforts to follow
medication, diet, and therapy plans. Your family may
need to help care for you at home.

You can expect us to help you identify sources of
follow-up care and to let you know if our hospital has a
financial interest in any referrals. As long as you agree
that we can share information about your care with
them, we will coordinate our activities with your
caregivers outside the hospital. You can also expect to
receive information and, where possible, training about
the self-care you will need when you go home.

Help with your bill and filing insurance claims. Our
staff will file claims for you with health care insurers or
other programs such as Medicare and Medicaid. They
also will help your doctor with needed documentation.
Hospital bills and insurance coverage are often confus-

ing. If you have questions about your bill, contact our business office. If you need help understanding your insurance coverage or health plan, start with your insurance company or health benefits manager. If you do not have health coverage, we will try to help you and your family find financial help or make other arrangements. We need your help with collecting needed information and other requirements to obtain coverage or assistance.

While you are here, you will receive more detailed notices about some of the rights you have as a hospital patient and how to exercise them. We are always interested in improving. If you have questions, comments, or concerns, please contact _____.

The Patient Care Partnership: Understanding Expectations, Rights and Responsibilities can be downloaded from *http://www.aha.org* in several languages including Arabic, Chinese, Russian, and Spanish.

In addition to general rights for general patients, all sorts of highly specialized subgroups have their own lists of rights: the disabled, the retarded, the pregnant, the dying, ad infinitum.

The American Nurses Association protects patients by spelling out nurses' responsibilities in a code of ethics, as shown here.

AMERICAN NURSES ASSOCIATION CODE OF ETHICS FOR NURSES

1. The nurse, in all professional relationships, practices with compassion and respect for the inherent dignity, worth and uniqueness of every individual, unrestricted by considerations of social or economic status, personal attributes, or the nature of health problems.

2. The nurse's primary commitment is to the patient, whether an individual, family, group, or community
3. The nurse promotes, advocates for, and strives to protect the health, safety, and rights of the patient.
4. The nurse is responsible and accountable for individual nursing practice and determines the appropriate delegation of tasks consistent with the nurse's obligation to provide optimum patient care.
5. The nurse owes the same duties to self as to others, including the responsibility to preserve integrity and safety, to maintain competence, and to continue personal and professional growth.
6. The nurse participates in establishing, maintaining, and improving healthcare environments and conditions of employment conducive to the provision of quality health care and consistent with the values of the profession through individual and collective action.
7. The nurse participates in the advancement of the profession through contributions to practice, education, administration, and knowledge development.
8. The nurse collaborates with other health professionals and the public in promoting community, national, and international efforts to meet health needs.
9. The profession of nursing, as represented by associations and their members, is responsible for articulating nursing values, for maintaining the integrity of the profession and its practice, and for shaping social policy.

Reprinted with permission from the American Nurses Association. *Code of Ethics for Nurses with Interpretive Statements*, Washington, DC: American Nurses Publishing, American Nurses Foundation/American Nurses Association, 2001.

Nursing students have written their own code of conduct. Here it is.

NATIONAL STUDENT NURSES ASSOCIATION CODE OF ACADEMIC AND CLINICAL CONDUCT

PREAMBLE

Students of nursing have a responsibility to society in learning the academic theory and clinical skills needed to provide nursing care. The clinical setting presents unique challenges and responsibilities while caring for human beings in a variety of health care environments.

The Code of Academic and Clinical Conduct is based on an understanding that to practice nursing as a student is an agreement to uphold the trust which society has placed in us. The statements of the Code provide guidance for the nursing student in the personal development of an ethical foundation and need not be limited strictly to the academic or clinical environment but can assist in the holistic development of the person.

A CODE FOR NURSING STUDENTS

As students are involved in the clinical and academic environments we believe that ethical principles are a necessary guide to professional development. Therefore within these environments we:

1. Advocate for the rights of all clients.
2. Maintain client confidentiality.

3. Take appropriate action to ensure the safety of clients, self, and others.
4. Provide care for the client in a timely, compassionate and professional manner.
5. Communicate client care in a truthful, timely and accurate manner.
6. Actively promote the highest level of moral and ethical principles and accept responsibility for our actions.
7. Promote excellence in nursing by encouraging lifelong learning and professional development.
8. Treat others with respect and promote an environment that respects human rights, values and choice of cultural and spiritual beliefs.
9. Collaborate in every reasonable manner with the academic faculty and clinical staff to ensure the highest quality of client care
10. Use every opportunity to improve faculty and clinical staff understanding of the learning needs of nursing students.
11. Encourage faculty, clinical staff, and peers to mentor nursing students.
12. Refrain from performing any technique or procedure for which the student has not been adequately trained.
13. Refrain from any deliberate action or omission of care in the academic or clinical setting that creates unnecessary risk of injury to the client, self, or others.
14. Assist the staff nurse or preceptor in ensuring that there is full disclosure and that proper authorizations are obtained from clients regarding any form of treatment or research.
15. Abstain from the use of alcoholic beverages or any substances in the academic and clinical setting that impair judgment.

16. Strive to achieve and maintain an optimal level of personal health.
17. Support access to treatment and rehabilitation for students who are experiencing impairments related to substance abuse and mental or physical health issues.
18. Uphold school policies and regulations related to academic and clinical performance, reserving the right to challenge and critique rules and regulations as per school grievance policy.

Reprinted with permission from the National Student Nurses Association, copyright 2001.

Nursing wants to do more than conform to the letter of the law: we also want to conform to the spirit of the law. We take our responsibility for the rights of others very seriously.

As nurses, we are so involved in protecting the rights of others that we often forget we have rights of our own. Perhaps that is why my list of "Ten Basic Rights for Nurses in the Health Professions" attracts so much attention.

1. You have the right to be treated with respect.
2. You have the right to a reasonable workload.
3. You have the right to an equitable wage.
4. You have the right to determine your own priorities.
5. You have the right to ask for what you want.
6. You have the right to refuse without making excuses or feeling guilty.
7. You have the right to make mistakes and be responsible for them.
8. You have the right to give and receive information as a professional.

9. You have the right to act in the best interest of the patient.
10. You have the right to be human.

It is not the rights themselves, but the very idea that nurses *have* rights, that is novel.

As a nursing student, you may be surprised to find that you have rights, too. For example, you have the right to see your educational records and to challenge information that you believe is inaccurate. Your records are to be kept private. With the exception of the registrar and your current instructor, no one should have access to your files without your permission. These rights are not at the discretion of the school but are legislated by Congress (Buckley Amendment). As expressed by the National Student Nurses' Association (NSNA):

"Every member of a nursing school must be held accountable for his/her action, be it an instructor, administrator or a student. NSNA believes that every school of nursing should have a written agreement between its students, faculty and administration."

This may be a good time to check into student rights on your campus. Rights are usually tucked away among the written rules, regulations, and requirements. They should include protection from capricious grading, incompetent instructors, and unsafe environments and should also provide specific guidelines for grievance procedures. To drive defensively you should know your rights long before you have to use them.

Even when rights are carefully spelled out, however, we know that there is a big difference between conforming to the letter of the law and conforming to the spirit of the law. Take the example of "informed consent." This is a paper that patients are asked to sign before surgery or treatment is undertaken. The document was developed to protect patients' rights. The intent was to make sure physicians instructed patients about their diagnoses, alternate treatments available, and potential risks or complications as well as potential benefits.

If you read consent forms from your local health care institutions, you will quickly see that they are written in terms only physicians and lawyers can understand. You will not be surprised to learn that (a) many patients think they have to sign and (b) the vast majority think the purpose is to protect physicians' rights, not their own.

By obtaining the patient's signature, the physician has "consent." He or she has conformed to the letter of the law. If the patient is truly "informed," then the doctor has conformed to the spirit of the law as well.

Most of us want to live up to the spirit of the law. All of us have to live up to the letter of the law if we want to maintain licensure and avoid litigation.

Until recently, nurses were seldom named as defendants in lawsuits. There were two reasons for this. First, nurses' salaries were so low that it literally did not pay to sue us. Second, nurses were assumed to be merely carrying out orders. We were not held accountable.

Today, we find nurses named in lawsuits right along with doctors and hospitals because our salaries have risen substantially and because nurses now carry malpractice insurance. That makes us profitable targets. In addition, nurses are no longer seen as robots mechanically carrying out doctors' orders. The law perceives us as fully functioning professionals and holds us responsible for our actions and for our failure to act. In fact, the law requires nurses to exercise more judgment than some physicians, administrators, or nurses may deem acceptable.

The legal implications of nursing care are so complex that whole books are devoted to the subject. Professional journals frequently run articles dealing with legal issues in nursing, and many have regular columns on the subject. Law has become a popular graduate school option for nurses, and the number of nurse-attorneys is growing rapidly.

To avoid the courtroom you must take a road that is paved with paperwork: charting, care plans, anecdotal notes, incident reports, and discharge summaries. Although paper-work is time-consuming, it should never be treated as trivial.

Donna Lee Guarriello, a nurse-attorney, provides a graphic illustration of the importance of paperwork. The case involved a young woman who had a cerebral hemorrhage and became permanently paralyzed after the birth of her first child. Initially, Guarriello intended to name the nurse together with two physicians in the lawsuit. After all, the nurse had spent 8 hours caring for the patient. During that time the patient's condition had steadily deteriorated. Apparently, the nurse had been negligent.

After reading the nurse's notes, however, the attorney decided not to sue her. According to the chart, the nurse had repeatedly tried to get proper attention and treatment for the patient. She had phoned the attending physician, suggesting that he transfer the patient to intensive care. He refused. She contacted her supervisor. When the attending physician did not come to the hospital and did not return her subsequent phone calls, she arranged for another obstetrician and a resident to see the patient. Unfortunately, they refused to countermand the orders of the attending physician.

Everything was thoroughly, objectively, and profes-sionally documented in the patient's chart. The nurse had not been negligent—quite the contrary. Paperwork did not help the patient, but it did save the nurse.

Always remember: defensive driving begins and ends with paperwork. When it comes to documenting patient care, pay close attention to your instructor. Don't waste time com-plaining about the amount of paperwork involved in nursing. Learn to do it efficiently and effectively. Your professional life may depend on it.

*"The illiterate in the 21st century will not be those who cannot read
and write but those who cannot learn, unlearn, and relearn."*
—Alvin Toffler

*"The reason why worry kills more people than work
is that more people worry than work."*
—Robert Frost

*"So many gods, so many creeds,
So many paths that wind and wind,
When just the art of being kind
Is all this sad world needs."*
—Ella Wheeler Wilcox

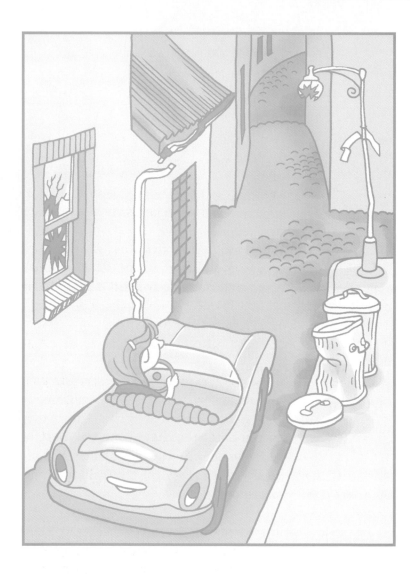

27

Street Smart

"Start each day with a smile and get it over with."
—W. C. Fields

You are traveling through a tough neighborhood. People here are sick and angry. And that's just the faculty! You have the staff and patients to deal with, too. What a shame everyone seems to gang up on students. You would swear no one remembered what it was like to be the new kid on the block.

Don't they remember what it was like to be a student? Yes, they do. They remember exactly what it was like. Most went through hell and high water to become nurses. Many are still convinced that it is the only way to initiate you into the profession. Before you can be a member, you have to prove your mettle. You have to show that you can stand up and take it like a nurse.

The only way to become part of any gang is to pay your dues. In nursing that means working together shoulder to shoulder, 40 hours a week, 50 weeks a year, for years and years. So when you enter the clinical setting, don't be surprised to feel like an outsider. You are an outsider. You are not part of the gang. If you are lucky, the staff will treat you like a guest. If you are unlucky, they will treat you like a trespasser.

Your instructor may or may not be part of the gang. Some faculty members have joint appointments, meaning they are employed by both the educational and the health care institutions. They have real-life responsibilities for both the clinical unit and the classroom.

Most instructors, however, have a sole employer: the school. Consequently, their status in the clinical unit may be almost equivalent to that of a student. Some instructors are warmly welcomed; others are barely tolerated. Given enough time and effort, faculty can earn a place in the gang. If your instructor has done so, count yourself lucky.

Nursing service and nursing education are often at odds. Each has a different mission, and sometimes they appear to be at cross purposes. Education strives for the ideal, whereas service must struggle with what is real.

For all practical purposes, you and your instructor are just passing through. The staff lives here. This is their turf, hard-fought and hard-won on a daily basis.

If you want to survive in this neighborhood, do not criticize the staff. Over the years, you will learn that there is a big difference between being book smart and being street smart.

To pave the way for the best possible clinical experience, you not only need to *give* a good first impression, you also need to *get* a good first impression.

GETTING A GOOD FIRST IMPRESSION

Unfortunately, every hospital is different, and every unit in every hospital is different. Just when you begin to feel comfortable in one clinical setting, you must rotate to another. Each new rotation begins with orientation—a rapid tour accompanied by a continuous stream of rules, regulations, policies, and preferences.

By the end of the tour, some students are so anxious that they can no longer tell a crash cart from a laundry cart. Their senses are jammed by the sights, sounds, and smells of the unit. Instead of reducing their anxiety, orientation seems to accentuate it.

If orientation gives you a headache instead of a head start, you may want to make a preorientation visit to the facility and to the unit to which you are assigned. Many students recommend visiting your new clinical setting a few days early. To get a general feeling of the place, they suggest you sit in the lobby, spend time in the patient waiting areas, eat in the cafeteria, and just ride the elevators. Make a mental map of the way to your unit, the nursing office, the major departments, laboratories, and clinics. Students recommend visiting your specific unit during the evening shift because it is usually less hectic than the day shift. Whatever time of day you choose, you are cautioned to avoid change-of-shift periods.

GIVING A GOOD FIRST IMPRESSION

Make sure you arrive at the clinical unit clean, pressed, and appropriately dressed. Wear your name tag and look like you mean business. The more professional you look, the more professional courtesy will be extended to you.

Stand tall and walk confidently. Look people in the eye. Smile. Be energetic but not hyperactive. Control nervous gestures such as cracking your knuckles or twisting your hair.

Introduce yourself and ask for the person in charge. Give your name, rank, and serial number. State your purpose and ask permission to enter the unit.

"I'm Sherry Jackson, a second-year student, and I'll be in this unit beginning Monday. Would it be OK if I looked around a little? I'd like to get my bearings before orientation."

If you want to get along with the gang, always show respect for their territory and their time. Remember the staff nurses' names. Call them by the title they prefer. Be friendly. Be sincere.

Let the staff do most of the talking. Be a good listener. Encourage them to talk about themselves and their professional experiences. You can learn a lot vicariously.

Ask their advice. Respect their opinions. Avoid arguing, criticizing, or complaining.

Get them to reminisce about their student days. They have some wonderful tales to tell. Listening to their war stories will reassure you about the future. If they survived, so can you. Recalling their past may also make them more sensitive to your present needs.

Always be ready to do a little more than required. Volunteer to give a hand without being asked. Say please and thank you. Common courtesy is all too uncommon.

PATIENTS PLEASE

Often, first impressions are formed even before you meet your patient. If you spend too much time studying the chart before going to his room, you may picture him as a series of problems, not as a person. If a staff member says, "So you're the one who got stuck with Mr. Elmers," you will have a much different first impression than if you are told, "Mr. Elmers is a terrific fellow. You are going to enjoy caring for him." Try to suspend judgment. Realize that first impressions or second-hand impressions may be more harmful than helpful.

The approaches that you used to make a good first impression on the staff can also help you make a good first impression on the patient—for example, dressing appropriately, looking professional, and controlling nervous gestures.

Before entering the patient's room, knock. Ask permission to enter. Respect what precious little turf the patient has.

Focus on the patient instead of on his tubes, dressings, or machinery. Look him in the eye. Pull up a chair and sit down. Introduce yourself and ask what name he prefers to be called. Tell him who you are and when you will be caring for him.

Before you leave, ask if he has any questions or if there is anything you can do for him. A simple act such as making sure the call bell is within reach, fetching fresh water, dialing the phone, fluffing the pillows, or finding out when he is scheduled for surgery can win him over.

HEARING WITH YOUR EYES

Street-smart students know that body language often contradicts verbal language. A patient winces yet says, "I'm fine." The head nurse says, "Welcome to 4 West," but her arms are folded tightly across her chest and her body is rigid.

Learning to listen with your eyes as well as your ears helps you interpret what is happening more accurately. By studying nonverbal communication, you will learn how to read people.

For example, did you know that leaning your head on one hand indicates interest, but leaning on both hands indicates boredom? Did you know that crossed arms are a sign of a closed mind, that locked ankles indicate worry or uncertainty, that a hand covering the mouth shows a lack of confidence and a reluctance to talk? Did you know that when people lie they tend to have rapid eye movements, lick their lips, rub their eyes, or scratch nervously?

As you learn more about body language, you will understand why it is not so much what you say but how you say it that counts. You observe one doctor who calls, "How are you?" from the doorway and another who goes to the bedside, touches the patient's shoulder, and asks the same question. The words are identical, but the effect is totally different. Which doctor really cares about the answer? Which doctor is going to get the more accurate response?

When trying to make a good impression, you choose your words carefully. Make the same careful choices when it comes to appearance, posture, and gestures. Actions do speak louder than words. Just ask any street-smart student.

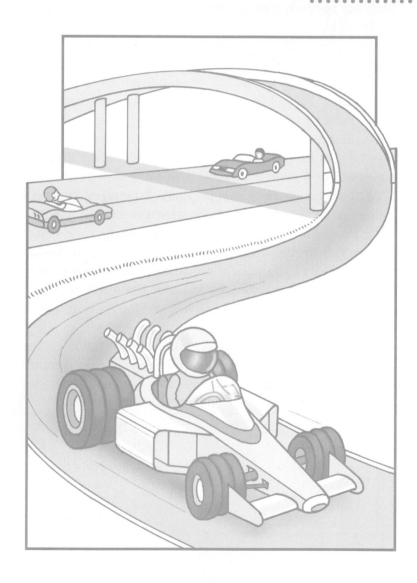

28

Life in the Fast Lane

"Now, here, you see, it takes all the running you can do, to keep in the same place. If you want to get somewhere else, you must run at least twice as fast as that!"
—Lewis Carroll, *Through the Looking Glass*

Well, it's time for one last lap around the track. And the last lap may be the hardest. *"People told me each year got easier—not true! Each year is harder."*

If you are approaching your final year, you may appreciate these tips from students who were only days away from graduation. To prepare for that last go-round, they suggest you:

"Spend the summer reviewing *everything* you've covered."

"Get all nonessentials (anything that doesn't pertain to school) out of the way before entering that last year."

"Get a summer job in a hospital. That experience will help you make the most of your last year."

"Try to identify your niche in nursing and request clinical experience in that area."

At the beginning of your final year, most students say, "really kick it into high gear" and "give it all you've got!"

"Try to get every possible experience. Keep in mind how quickly a year goes. Get everything you can NOW!"

"Challenge *yourself*. Don't worry about grades."

"Keep your eye on your goal. Make every moment count."

"Quit your job. Don't work if at all possible. Focus all your energies on learning anything and everything."

"Read every nursing journal you can get your hands on."

"Join all the professional organizations and clubs you can."

"Attend in-service programs at the hospital whenever possible."

"Get involved. Become politically, financially, and professionally informed—do not have tunnel vision about your profession."

"Work hard ... it will all be over soon."

Other students suggest you ease up a bit on the accelerator:

"Relax! This is what you've been waiting for. You're about to accomplish a very important goal."

"Enjoy your last year. When it's over, you're going to miss it."

"Relax. You know more than you think you do."

"Take time out to reflect on all you've accomplished."

No matter how tough things get, don't quit! A student from Texas said, "If I can make it, you can make it!" She's right. Every year about 80,000 nursing students "make it."

You might as well be one of them. So ...

"Don't give up! Keep fighting!"

"Hang on!"

"Think POSITIVE!"

"Keep swimming, Babe, the shore is in sight!"

The good news is that you are about to graduate. That's also the bad news. If you graduate, you have to face state board examinations. The mere mention of state boards—the final to end all finals—produces something akin to mass hysteria. These near-graduates suggest that you not become obsessed by state boards but rather prepare for them confidently and systematically.

"First things first. Concentrate on school."

"Write for information on state board testing dates."

"Buy a review book and pledge to spend 15 minutes a day with it."

"Form a group specifically to study for boards."

"Don't panic. Your instructors will help you. After all, if you don't look good, they don't look good."

"Enroll in a review course. They are available." (A list of Mosby's review books and courses appears in Appendix G.)

As graduation approaches and attentions shift to finding a job, seniors advise you to:

"Start surveying employment opportunities early. Read the nursing career guides as well as the classified ads in newspapers."

"Form a job-search club. Critique each other's résumés. Discuss local and national career opportunities."

"Talk with recruiters and write to as many hospitals as possible for information. Xerox anything you get, and share it with classmates. You're all in this together."

"Look for a mentor. See if there's an opportunity to work alongside a nurse you admire."

"Look for a hospital that offers an extensive, comprehensive internship program for new grads."

"Talk to last year's graduates and find out how they like their jobs. Ask them for suggestions. Is there anything they wish they had done differently in their senior year?"

"Remember, nursing is loaded with possibilities. Keep an open mind about specialization, new directions, and professional goals. You may be surprised!"

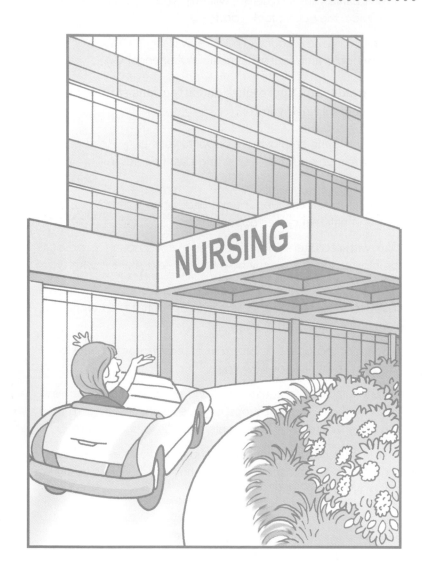

29

Are We There Yet?

"O Captain! my Captain! our fearful trip is done!
The ship has weather'd every wreck,
the prize we sought is won,
The port is near; the bells I hear;
The people all exulting."
—Walt Whitman, *O Captain! My Captain!*

O nce you have graduated and passed the state board exams, you have arrived. And yet, the journey is just beginning.

You surrender your learner's permit and pick up a professional license. One moment you are a thoroughly experienced student. The next moment you are a thoroughly inexperienced professional.

But, if you have gotten this far, YOU CAN DO ANYTHING.

APPENDIXES

A   Common Prefixes and Suffixes Used in Nursing

B   Sources of Scholarships and Loans

C   State Nurses Associations

D   Canadian Nurses Associations

E   Specialty Nursing Organizations

F   U.S. State and Territorial Boards of Nursing

G   Resources for NCLEX® Review Available from Mosby/Elsevier

Common Prefixes and Suffixes Used in Nursing

PREFIXES	MEANING
a-, an-	without, not
ab-	away from
ad-	to, toward
adeno-	gland
aero-	air
ambi-	around
amphi-	about, on both sides, both
ampho-	both
ana-	up, back, again, excessive
angio-	vessel
ano-	anus
ante-	before, forward
anti-	against, counteracting
ap-, apo-	from, separation
arterio-	artery
arthro-	joint
bi-	double
bili-	bile
bio-	life
bis-	two
brachio-	arm
brady-	slow
broncho-	bronchus
cardio-	heart
cata-	down, under, lower, against
cepha-, cephalo-	head
cerebro-	cerebrum
cervico-	neck
chole-	gall, bile
cholecysto-	gallbladder
chondro-	cartilage
circum-	around
co-	together

PREFIXES	MEANING
com-, con-	with, together
contra-	opposite, against
costo-	ribs
cranio-	head
cyto-	cell
cysto-	bladder
de-	away from
demi-	half
derm-, derma-	skin
dia-	between, through, apart, across, completely
dis-	from
dorso-	back
dys	difficult, abnormal
e-, ex-, exo	out, away from
ec-	out from
ecto-	on outer side, situated on
electro-	related to electricity
em-, en-	in
encephal-	brain
endo-	within
entero-	intestines
epi-	upon, on
equi-	equal
eryth-	red
extra-	in addition to, outside of
ferro-	iron
fibro-	fiber
fore-	in front of, before
gastro-	stomach
glosso-	tongue
glyco-	sugar
hemi-	half
hemo-, hema-	blood
hepa-, hepato-	liver
histo-	tissue
homo-	same
hydro-	water
hyper-	high, excessive

PREFIXES	MEANING
hypo-	low, decreased
hyster-, hystero-	uterus
im-, in-	in, into, not
infra-	below
inter-	between
intra-	within
intro-	in, into, within
juxta-	near, close
laparo-	abdomen
laryngo-	larynx
latero-	side
leuk-	white
lympho-	lymph
macro-	large
mal-	poor, bad
mast, masto-	breast
medio-	middle
mega-	large, great
meno-	menses
meta-	beyond, after, change
micro-	small
mono-	single
multi-	many
myelo-	spinal cord, bone marrow
myo-	muscle
naso-	nose
neo-	new
nephro-	kidney
neuro-	nerve
nitro-	nitrogen
noct-	night
non-	not
ob-	in front of, against
oculo-	eye
odonto-	tooth
oophoro-	ovary
ophthalmo-	eye
opistho-	behind, backward
orchio-, orchido-	testes

PREFIXES	MEANING
ortho-	straight, normal
os-	mouth, bone
osteo-	bone
oto-	ear
ovario-	ovary
pan-	all
para-	beside, along with
path-	disease
ped-	child, foot
per-	by, through
peri-	around
pharyngo-	pharynx
phlebo-	vein
photo-	light
pneumo-	air, lungs
pod-	foot
poly-	many, much
post-	after, behind
pre-, pro-	before, in front of
proct-, procto-	rectum
pseudo-	false
psych-	mind
pyo-	pus
pyro-	fever
quadri-	four
radio-	radiation
re-	back, again
reno-	kidney
retro-	backward
rhino-	nose
sacro-	sacrum
sclero-	hard, hardening
semi-	half
spleno-	spleen
steno-	narrowing, construction
sterno-	sternum
sub-	under
super-, supra-	above, excess
sym-, syn-	together

PREFIXES	MEANING
tachy-	fast
teno-	tendon
thyro-	thyroid
trache-	trachea
trans-	throughout, across
tri-	three
ultra-	beyond
un-	not, reversal
uni-	one
uretero-	ureter
urethro-	urethra
uro-	urine
vaso-	blood vessel
veno-	vein

SUFFIXES	MEANING
-able	able to
-algia	pain
-cele	swelling, tumor
-centesis	surgical puncture
-cide	destructive, killing
-cule	little
-cyte	cell
-ectasia	expansion, dilation
-ectomy	excision
-emia	blood
-esis	action
-form	shaped like
-genesis	origin, formation
-graph	writing
-iasis, -ism	condition
-itis	inflammation
-ize	to treat
-lith	stone
-lysis	disintegration, dissolution
-malacia	softening
-megaly	enlargement
-meter	measuring instrument
-oid	resemblance, likeness

SUFFIXES	MEANING
-oma	tumor
-opathy, -pathy	any disease of
-orrhaphy	surgical repair
-osis	disease
-ostomy, -stomy	to form an opening
-otomy, -tomy	incision into
-penia	deficiency, decrease
-phage	ingesting
-phobia	fear

Sources of Scholarships and Loans

Johnson & Johnson has created a wonderful website to help promote careers in nursing. Go to *http://www.discovernursing.com,* and you will find lots of valuable information including *hundreds of scholarships* available to nursing students.

Don't forget to check with the financial aid office at your school. Then check out this list of state higher education agencies. They have information on education programs, colleges and universities, financial aid assistance programs, grants, scholarships, continuing education programs, and career opportunities.

Alabama Commission on Higher Education
PO Box 302000
Montgomery, AL 36130-2000
http://www.ache.state.al.us

Alaska Commission on Postsecondary Education
3030 Vintage Blvd
Juneau, AK 99801-7100
http://www.state.ak.us/acpe

Arizona Commission for Postsecondary Education
2020 North Central Ave, Suite 275
Phoenix, AZ 85004-4503
http://www.acpe.asu.edu

Arkansas Department of Higher Education
114 East Capitol
Little Rock, AR 72201-3818
http://www.adhe.arknet.edu

California Student Aid Commission
PO Box 419027
Rancho Cordova, CA 95741-9027
http://www.csac.ca.gov

Colorado Commission on Higher Education
1380 Lawrence St, Suite 1200
Denver, CO 80204
http://www.state.co.us/cc hedir/hecche.html

Connecticut Department of Higher Education
61 Woodland St
Hartford, CT 06105-1310
http://www.ctdhe.org

Delaware Higher Education Commission
Carvel State Office Building, Fifth Floor
Wilmington, DE 19801
http://www.doe.state.de.us/high-ed

District of Columbia Dept. of Human Services
Office of Postsecondary Education, Research, and Assistance
Suite 401
2100 Martin Luther King, Jr. Ave SE
Washington, DC 20020

Florida Office of Student Financial Assistance
Department of Education
Florida Education Center
Tallahassee, FL 32399

Georgia Student Finance Authority
State Loans and Grants Division
Suite 200
2082 East Exchange Pl
Tucker, GA 30084
http://www.gsfc.org

Hawaii State Postsecondary Education Commission
2444 Dole St, Room 209
Honolulu, HI 96822-2302
http://www.hern.hawaii.
edu/hern

Idaho Board of Education
PO Box 83720
Boise, ID 83720-0027
http://www.sde.state.id.
ua/osbe/board.htm

Illinois Student Assistance Commission
1755 Lake Cook Rd
Deerfield, IL 60015-5209
http://www.isac-
online.org

State Student Assistance Commission of Indiana
150 West Market St,
Suite 500
Indianapolis, IN
46204-2811
http://www.in.gov/ssaci

Iowa College Student Aid Commission
200 10th St,
Fourth Floor
Des Moines, IA 50309
http://www.state.ia.us/
collegeaid

Kansas Board of Regents
700 SW Harrison
Suite 1410
Topeka, KS 66603-3760
http://www.
kansasregents.org

Kentucky Higher Education Assistance Authority
1050 U.S. Highway 127 S
Frankfort, KY
40601-4323
http://www.kheaa.com

Louisiana Office of Student Financial Assistance
PO Box 91202
Baton Rouge, LA
70821-9202
http://www.osfa.state.
la.us

Maine Education Assistance Division
Finance Authority of
Maine
5 Community Dr
Augusta, ME 04332-0949
http://www.famemaine.
com

Maryland Higher Education Commission
Jeffrey Building
16 Francis St
Annapolis, MD 21401-
1781
http://www.mhec.state.
md.us

Massachusetts Board of Higher Education
One Ashburton Pl,
Room 1401
Boston, MA 02109
http://www.mass.edu

Massachusetts Higher Education Information Center
Boston Public Library
700 Boylston St
Boston, MA 02116
http://www.adinfo.org

Michigan Higher Education Assistance Authority
Office of Scholarships
and Grants
PO Box 30462
Lansing, MI 48909-7962
http://www.
MI-StudentAid.org

Minnesota Higher Education Services Office
1450 Energy Park Dr,
Suite 350
Saint Paul, MN
55108-5227
http://www.mheso.state.
mn.us/cfdocs/web
directory/index.cfm

Mississippi Office of Student Financial Aid
3825 Ridgewood Rd
Jackson, MS 39211-6453
http://www.ihl.state.
ms.us

Missouri Department of Higher Education
3515 Amazonas Dr
Jefferson City, MO
65109-5717
http://www.gov.state.
mo.us/ boards/cgi?
FUNCTION=
MAIN&
BOARD
=CBHE

Montana University System
2500 Broadway
Helena, MT 59620-3103
http://www.montana.
edu/wwwoche

Nebraska Coordinating Commission for Postsecondary Education
140 North Eighth St, Suite 300
Lincoln, NE 68509-2886
http://www.ccpe.state.ne.us/PublicDoc/CCPE/Default.asp

Nevada Financial Aid Office
University of Nevada-Reno
Room 300 TSSC
Reno, NV 89557

New Hampshire Postsecondary Education Commission
2 Industrial Park Dr
Concord, NH 03301-8512
http://www.state.nh.us/postsecondary

New Jersey Higher Education Student Assistance Authority
Quakerbridge Plaza, Building 4
Trenton, NJ 08625-0540
http://www.hesaa.org

New Mexico Commission on Higher Education
1068 Cerrillos Rd
Santa Fe, NM 87501
http://www.nmche.org

New York State Higher Education Services Corp.
99 Washington Ave
Albany, NY 12255
http://www.hesc.com

North Carolina State Education Assistance Authority
PO Box 13663
Research Triangle Park, NC 27709-3663
http://www.neseaa.edu

North Dakota University System
North Dakota Student Financial Assistance Program
Department 215
600 East Boulevard Ave
Bismarck, ND 58505-0230
http://www.nodak.edu

Ohio Board of Regents
State Grants and Scholarships Department
PO Box 182452
Columbus, OH 43218-2452
http://www.regents.state.oh.us/sgs

Oklahoma State Regents for Higher Education
Oklahoma Guaranteed Student Loan Program
655 Research Pkwy, Suite 200
Oklahoma, OK 73104
http://www.okhighered.org

Oregon Student Assistance Commission
1500 Valley River Dr, Suite 100
Eugene, OR 97401
http://www.osac.state.or.us

Pennsylvania Higher Education Assistance Agency
1200 North Seventh St
Harrisburg, PA 17102-1444
http://www.pheaa.org

Rhode Island Higher Education Assistance Authority
560 Jefferson Blvd
Warwick, RI 02886
http://www.riheaa.org

Rhode Island Office of Higher Education
301 Promenade St
Providence, RI 20908-5748
http://www.ribghe.org/riohe.htm

South Carolina Tuition Grants Agency
411 Keenan Building
Columbia, SC 29211

South Dakota Board of Regents
306 East Capitol Ave
Pierre, SD 57501
http://www.ris.sdbor.edu

Tennessee Higher Education Commission
Parkway Towers, Suite 1900
404 James Robertson Pkwy
Nashville, TN 37243-6230
http://www.state.tn.us/thec

Texas Higher Education Coordinating Board
PO Box 12788
Austin, TX 78711
http://www.thecb.state.tx.us

Utah State Board of Regents
Three Triad Center,
  Suite 550
355 West North Temple
Salt Lake City, UT
  84180-1205
http://www.utahsbr.edu

Vermont Student Assistance Corporation
Chaplain Mill
1 Main St, Fourth Floor
Winooski, VT 05404-2601
http://www.vsac.org

State Council of Higher Education for Virginia
James Monroe Building,
  Ninth Floor
101 North 14th St
Richmond, VA 23219
http://www.schev.edu

Washington State Higher Education Coordinating Board
917 Lakeridge Way
Olympia, WA 98504-3430
http://www.hecb.wa.gov

West Virginia Higher Education Policy Commission
1018 Kanawha Blvd,
  East
Charleston, WV 25301
http://www.hepc.wvnet.
  edu

Wisconsin Higher Educational Aids Board
131 West Wilson St,
  Room 902
Madison, WI 53707-7885
http://www.heab.state.
  wi.us

Wyoming Community College Commission
2020 Carey Ave
Cheyenne, WY 82002
http://www.commission.
  wcc.edu

State Nurses Associations

American Nurses Association
8515 Georgia Ave, Suite 400
Silver Spring, MD 20910
http://www.
nursingworld.org

Alabama State Nurses' Association
360 North Hull St
Montgomery, AL 36104-3658
http://www.
alabamanurses.org

Alaska Nurses Association
2207 East Tudor Rd, Suite 34
Anchorage, AK 99507-1069
http://www.aknurse.org

Arizona Nurses Association
1850 E Southern Ave, Suite #1
Tempe, AZ 85282
http://www.aznurse.org

Arkansas Nurses Association
1401 W Capitol Ave, Suite 155
Little Rock, AR 72201
http://www.arna.org

ANA-California
1121 L St, Suite 409
Sacramento, CA 95814
http://www.anacalifornia.
org

Colorado Nurses Association
1221 South Clarkson St, Suite 205
Denver, CO 80210
http://www.nurses-co.org

Connecticut Nurses Association
337 Research Pkwy, Suite 2D
Meriden, CT 06450
http://www.ctnurses.org

Delaware Nurses Association
2644 Capitol Trail, Suite 330
Newark, DE 19711
http://www.denurses.org

District of Columbia Nurses Association, Inc.
5100 Wisconsin Ave, NW, Suite 306
Washington, DC 20016
http://www.dcna.org

Federal Nurses Association
8515 Georgia Ave, Suite 400
Silver Spring, MD 20910
http://www.nursingworld.
org/FedNA

Florida Nurses Association
PO Box 536985
Orlando, FL 32853-6985
http://www.floridanurse.
org

Georgia Nurses Association
3032 Briarcliff Rd NE
Atlanta, GA 30329-2655
http://www.georgia
nurses.org

Guam Nurses Association
PO Box CG
Hagatna, Guam 96932

Hawaii Nurses Association
677 Ala Moana Blvd, Suite 301
Honolulu, HI 96813
http://www.hawaiinurses.
org

Idaho Nurses Association
200 North 4th St, Suite 20
Boise, ID 83702-6001
http://www.nursingworld.
org/snas/id

Illinois Nurses Association
105 West Adams St, Suite 2101
Chicago, IL 60603
http://www.illinoisnurses.
com

Indiana State Nurses Association
2915 North High School Rd
Indianapolis, IN 46224
http://www.indiananurses.
org

Iowa Nurses Association
1501 42nd St, Suite 471
West Des Moines, IA
  50266
http://www.iowanurses.
  org

Kansas State Nurses Association
1208 SW Tyler
Topeka, KS 66612-1735
http://www.nursingworld.
  org/snas/ks

Kentucky Nurses Association
1400 South First St
Louisville, KY 40201-
  2616
http://www.kentucky-
  nurses.org

Louisiana State Nurses Association
5800 One Perkins Pl,
  Suite 2-B
Baton Rouge, LA 70808
http://www.lsna.org

ANA-Maine
PO Box 3000, PMB #280
York, ME 03909
http://www.anamaine.org

Maryland Nurses Association
21 Governor's Ct,
  Suite 195
Baltimore, MD 21244
http://www.marylandrn.
  org

Massachusetts Association of Registered Nurses
PO Box 70668
Worcester, MA 01607-
  0688
http://www.marnonline.
  org

Michigan Nurses Association
2310 Jolly Oak Rd
Okemos, MI 48864-4599
http://www.minurses.org

Minnesota Nurses Association
1625 Energy Park Dr
St. Paul, MN 55108
http://www.mnnurses.
  org

Mississippi Nurses Association
31 Woodgreen Pl
Madison, MS 39110
http://www.msnurses.org

Missouri Nurses Association
1904 Bubba Ln
Jefferson City, MO
  65110-5228
http://www.missouri
  nurses.org

Montana Nurses Association
104 Broadway, Suite G-2
Helena, MT 59601
http://www.mtnurses.org

Nebraska Nurses Association
715 South 14th St
Lincoln, NE 68508
http://www.nursingworld
  .org/snas/ne

Nevada Nurses Association
PO Box 530399
Reno, NV 89533
http://www.nvnurses.org

New Hampshire Nurses Association
48 West St
Concord, NH 03301-3595
http://www.nhnurses.org

New Jersey State Nurses Association
1479 Pennington Rd
Trenton, NJ 08618-2661
http://www.njsna.org

New Mexico Nurses Association
PO Box 29658
Santa Fe, NM 87592-
  9658
http://www.nursingworld.
  org/snas/nm

New York State Nurses Association
11 Cornell Rd
Latham, NY 12110
http://www.nysna.org

North Carolina Nurses Association
103 Enterprise St
Raleigh, NC 27605
http://www.ncnurses.org

North Dakota Nurses Association
531 Airport Rd, Suite D
Bismarck, ND 58504-
  6107
http://www.ndna.org

Ohio Nurses Association
4000 East Main St
Columbus, OH 43213-
  2983
http://www.ohnurses.org

Oklahoma Nurses Association
6414 North Santa Fe,
  Suite A
Oklahoma City, OK
  73116
http://www.oknurses.com

Oregon Nurses Association
18765 SW Boones
    Ferry Rd
Tualatin, OR 97062
http://www.oregonrn.org

Pennsylvania State Nurses Association
2578 Interstate Dr,
    Suite 101
Harrisburg, PA 17110-
    9601
http://www.psnurses.org

Rhode Island State Nurses Association
550 S Water St,
    Unit 540B
Providence, RI 02903-
    4344
http://www.risnarn.org

South Carolina Nurses Association
1821 Gadsden St
Columbia, SC 29201
http://www.scnurses.org

South Dakota Nurses Association
116 N Euclid
Pierre, SD 57501-1015
http://www.nursing
    world.org/snas/sd

Tennessee Nurses Association
545 Mainstream Dr,
    Suite 405
Nashville, TN 37228-
    1201
http://www.tnaonline.org

Texas Nurses Association
7600 Burnet Rd,
    Suite 440
Austin, TX 78757-1292
http://www.texasnurses.
    org

Utah Nurses Association
4505 South Wasatch
    Blvd, #290
Salt Lake City, UT
    84124
http://www.utahnurses.
    org

Vermont State Nurses Association
100 Dorset St, Suite 13
South Burlington, VT
    05403-6241
http://www.uvm.edu/
    ~vsna

Virgin Islands State Nurses Association
PO Box 2339
Kings Hill
U.S. Virgin Islands
    00821-0583

Virginia Nurses Association
7113 Three Chopt Rd,
    Suite 204
Richmond, VA 23226
http://www.virginia
    nurses.com

Washington State Nurses Association
575 Andover Park West,
    Suite 101
Seattle, WA 98188-3321
http://www.wsna.org

West Virginia Nurses Association
100 Capitol St,
    Suite 1009
Charleston, WV 25301
http://www.wvnurses.org

Wisconsin Nurses Association
6117 Monona Dr
Madison, WI 53716
http://www.
    wisconsinnurses.org

Wyoming Nurses Association
Majestic Building,
    Room 305
PO Box 895
Casper, WY 82602-0895
http://www.wyonurse.
    org

Canadian Nurses Associations

Canadian Nurses Association
50 Driveway
Ottawa, Ontario K2P 1E2
http://www.can-nurses.ca

Canadian Nursing Students' Association
325-350 Albert St
Ottawa, Ontario K1R 1B1
http://www.cnsa.ca

Aboriginal Nurses Association of Canada
192 Bank St
Ottawa, Ontario K2P 1W8
http://www.anac.on.ca

The Alberta Association of Registered Nurses
11620 168th St
Edmonton, Alberta T5M 4A6
http://www.nurses.ab.ca

Association of Nurses of Prince Edward Island
17 Pownal St
Charlottetown, Prince Edward Island C1A 3V7

Association of Registered Nurses of Newfoundland
55 Military Rd, Box 6116
St. Johns, Newfoundland A1C 5X8
http://www.arnn.nf.ca

Canadian Association for the History of Nursing
University of Alberta
114 89th Ave
Edmonton, Alberta T6G 2M7
http://www.cahn-achn.ca/

The Canadian Intravenous Nurses Association
18 Wynford Dr, Suite 516
North York, Ontario M36 3S2
http://www.csotcina.com

Canadian Nurses Foundation
50 Driveway
Ottawa, Ontario K2P 1E2
http://www.can-nurses.cacnf

College of Nurses of Ontario
101 Davenport Rd
Toronto, Ontario M5R 3P1
http://www.cno.org

College of Registered Nurses of Nova Scotia
Suite 66, Barrington Tower
1894 Barrington St
Halifax, Nova Scotia B3J 2A8
http://www.rnans.ns.ca

Manitoba Association of Registered Nurses
647 Broadway
Winnipeg, Manitoba R3C 0X2
http://www.marn.nb.ca

Northwest Territories Registered Nurses Association
PO Box 2757
Yellowknife, Northwest Territories X0E 1H0
http://www.nwtrna.com

Nurse Association of New Brunswick
165 Regent St
Fredericton, New Brunswick E3B 3W5
http://www.nanb.nb.ca

Ontario Nurses' Association
85 Grenville St, Suite 400
Toronto, Ontario M5S 3A2
http://www.ona.org

Order of Nurses of the Province of Quebec
4200 Dorchester Blvd W
Montreal, Quebec H3Z 1V4
http://www.oiiq.org

Registered Nurses Association of British Columbia
2855 Arbutus St
Vancouver, British Columbia V6J 3Y8
http://www.rnabc.bc.ca

Registered Nurses Association of Ontario
438 University Ave, Suite 1600
Toronto, Ontario M5G 2K8
http://www.rnao.org

Saskatchewan Registered Nurses' Association
2066 Retallack St
Regina, Saskatchewan S4T 7X5
http://www.srna.org

United Nurses of Alberta
#900, 10611 98th Ave
Edmonton, Alberta T5K 2P7
http://www.una.ab.ca

Yukon Nurses Society
204-4133 4th Ave
Whitehorse, Yukon Y1A 3T3

Specialty Nursing Organizations

Academy of Medical-Surgical Nurses
E Holly Ave, Box 56
Pitman, NJ 08071-0056
http://www.
medsurgnurse.org

Air & Surface Transport Nurses Association
915 Lee St
Des Plaines, IL 60016-6569
http://www.astna.org

American Academy of Ambulatory Care Nursing
E Holly Ave, Box 56
Pitman, NJ 08071-0056
http://www.aaacn.org

American Academy of Nurse Practitioners
PO Box 12846
Austin, TX 78711
http://www.aanp.org

American Academy of Nursing
600 Maryland Ave SW
Suite 100 West
Washington, DC 20024-2571
http://www.nursingworld.
org/aan

American Academy of Wound Management
1255 23rd St NW,
Suite 200
Washington, DC 20037
http://www.aawm.org

American Assembly for Men in Nursing
c/o NYSNA
11 Cornell Rd
Latham, NY 12110-1499
http://www.aamn.org

American Association for the History of Nursing
PO Box 175
Lanoka Harbor, NJ 08734
http://www.aahn.org

American Association of Colleges of Nursing
1 Dupont Cir, NW,
Suite 530
Washington, DC 20036
http://www.aacn.nche.
edu

American Association of Critical-Care Nurses
101 Columbia
Aliso Viejo, CA 92656-1491
http://www.aacn.org

American Association of Diabetes Educators
100 W Monroe St,
4th Floor
Chicago, IL 60603-1901
http://www.aadenet.org

American Association of Legal Nurse Consultants
4700 W Lake Ave
Glenview, IL 60025
http://www.aalnc.org

The American Association of Managed Care Nurses, Inc.
4435 Waterfront Dr,
Suite 101
Glen Allen, VA 23060
http://www.aamcn.org

American Association of Neuroscience Nurses
4700 W Lake Ave
Glenview, IL 60025
http://www.aann.org

American Association of Nurse Anesthetists
222 S Prospect Ave
Park Ridge, IL 60068-4001
http://www.aana.com

The American Association of Nurse Attorneys
7794 Grow Dr
Pensacola, FL 32514
http://www.taana.org

American Association of Occupational Health Nurses, Inc.
2920 Brandywine Rd,
Suite 100
Atlanta, GA 30341
http://www.aaohn.org

American Association of Office Nurses
109 Kinderkamack Rd
Montvale, NJ 07645
http://www.aaon.org

American Association of Spinal Cord Nurses
75-20 Astoria Blvd
Jackson Heights, NY 11370
http://www.aascin.org

American Board of Nursing Specialties
4035 Running Springs
San Antonio, TX 78261
http://www.nursing-certification.org

American College of Nurse Midwives
8403 Colesville Rd, Suite 1550
Silver Spring, MD 20910
http://www.midwife.org

American College of Nurse Practitioners
503 Capitol Ct NE, #300
Washington, DC 20002
http://www.nurse.org/acnp

American Forensic Nurses
225 N El Cielo Rd, Suite 195
Palm Springs, CA 92262
http://www.amrn.com

American Holistic Nurses Association
PO Box 2130
Flagstaff, AZ 86003-2130
http://www.ahna.org

American Long Term & Sub Acute Nurses Association
PO Box 1304
Toms River, NJ 08753
http://www.alsna.com

American Nephrology Nurses' Association
E Holly Ave, Box 56
Pitman, NJ 08071-0056
http://www.annanurse.org

American Organization of Nurse Executives
1 N Franklin
Chicago, IL 60606
http://www.aone.org

American Psychiatric Nurses Association
1555 Wilson Blvd, Suite 602
Arlington, VA 22209
http://www.apna.org

American Society of Perianesthesia Nurses
10 Melrose Ave, Suite 110
Cherry Hill, NJ 08003-3696
http://www.aspan.org

American Radiological Nurses Association
820 Jorie Blvd
Oak Brook, IL 60523-2251
http://www.rsna.org

American Society for Long-Term Care Nurses
660 Lonely Cottage Dr
Upper Black Eddy, PA 18972-9313

American Society of Pain Management Nurses
7794 Grow Dr
Pensacola, FL 32514
http://www.aspmn.org

American Society of PeriAnesthesia Nurses
6900 Grove Rd
Thorofare, NJ 08060
http://www.aspan.org

American Society of Plastic and Reconstructive Surgical Nurses
E Holly Ave, Box 56
Pitman, NJ 08071-0056
http://www.asprsn.org

Association for Professionals in Infection Control and Epidemiology, Inc.
1275 K St NW, Suite 1000
Washington, DC 20005-4006

Association of Nurses in AIDS Care
11250 Roger Bacon Dr, Suite 8
Reston, VA 20190-5202
http://www.anacnet.org

Association of Pediatric Oncology Nurses
4700 W Lake Ave
Glenview, IL 60025
http://www.spon.org

Association of Perioperative Registered Nurses
2170 S Parker Rd, Suite 300
Denver, CO 80231-5711
http://www.aorn.org

Association of Rehabilitation Nurses
4700 W Lake Ave
Glenview, IL 60025-1485
http://www.rehabnurse.org

Association of Women's Health, Obstetric and Neonatal Nurses
2000 L St NW, Suite 740
Washington, DC 20036
http://www.awhonn.org

**Case Management
Society of America**
8201 Cantrell, Suite 230
Little Rock, AR 72227
http://www.cmsa.org

**Center for Nursing
Advocacy**
203 Churchwardens Rd
Baltimore, MD 21212-
2937
http://www.nursing-
advocacy.org

**Chi Eta Phi Sorority,
Inc.**
3029 Thirteenth St NW
Washington, DC 20009
http://www.chietaphi.com

**Emergency Nurses
Association**
915 Lee St
Des Plaines, IL 60016-
6569
http://www.ena.org

**Endocrine Nurses
Society**
4350 E West Hwy,
Suite 500
Bethesda, MD 20814-
4410
http://www.endo-
nurses.org

**Home Health Nurses
Association**
228 Seventh St SE
Washington, DC 20003
http://www.nahc.org/
hhna

**Hospice and Palliative
Nurses Association**
Penn Center West One,
Suite 229
Pittsburgh, PA 15276
http://www.hpna.org

Infusion Nurses Society
220 Norwood Park S
Norwood, MA 02062
http://www.ins1.org

**International Council
of Nurses**
3, Place Jean Marteau
1201-Geneva
Switzerland
http://www.icn.ch

**International Society
of Nurses in Genetics**
22593 West 15th St S
Newton, IA 50208-8500
http://www.isong.org

**International Transplant
Nurses Society**
1739 E Carson St,
Box 351
Pittsburgh, PA 15203-
1700
http://www.itns.org

**Intravenous Nurses
Society**
Fresh Pond Sq,
10 Fawcett St
Cambridge, MA 02138
http://www.ins1.org

**League of Intravenous
Therapy Education**
Empire Bldg, Suite 3
3001 Jacks Run Rd
White Oak, PA 15131
http://www.lite.org

**National Alliance of
Nurse Practitioners**
325 Pennsylvania Ave
SE, PMB 350
Washington, DC 20003-
1100

**National Association of
Clinical Nurse
Specialists**
3969 Green St
Harrisburg, PA 17110
http://www.nacns.org

**National Association of
Hispanic Nurses**
1501 16th St NW
Washington, DC 20036
http://www.nahnhq.org

**National Association of
Neonatal Nurses**
4700 W Lake Ave
Glenview, IL 60025-1485
http://www.nann.org

**National Association of
Nurse Massage
Therapists**
PO Box 820
Clarkdale, AZ 86324
http://www.member.aol.
com/nanmt1

**National Association of
Orthopaedic Nurses**
E Holly Ave, Box 56
Pitman, NJ 08071-0056
http://www.naon.
inurse. com

**National Association of
Pediatric Nurse
Associates &
Practitioners, Inc.**
1101 Kings Hwy N,
Suite 206
Cherry Hill, NJ 08034-
1912
http://www.napnap.org

**National Association of
School Nurses**
PO Box 1300
Scarborough, ME 04070-
1300
http://www.nasn.org

**National Association of
Vascular Access
Networks**
11417 S 700 East,
PMB 205
Draper, UT 84020
http://www.navannet.org

**National Black Nurses
Association, Inc.**
8630 Fenton St,
Suite 330
Silver Spring, MD 20910-
3803
http://www.nbna.org

National Coalition of Ethnic Minority Nurse Associations
6100 West Centinela Ave, Suite 378
Culver City, CA 90230
http://www.ncemna.org

National Council of State Boards of Nursing, Inc.
676 N St. Clair St, Suite 550
Chicago, IL 60611-2921
http://www.ncsbn.org

The National Federation for Specialty Nursing Organizations
E Holly Ave, Box 56
Pitman, NJ 08071
http://www.nfsno.org

National Federation of Licensed Practical Nurses, Inc.
893 U.S. Hwy 70 W, Suite 202
Garner, NC 27529
http://www.nflpn.org

National Gerontological Nursing Association
7794 Grow Dr
Pensacola, FL 32514
http://www.ngna.org

National League for Nursing
61 Broadway, 33rd Floor
New York, NY 10006
http://www.nln.org

National Nurses Society on Addictions
4101 Lake Boone Trail, Suite 201
Raleigh, NC 27067
http://www.nnsa.org

National Nursing Staff Development Organization
7794 Grow Dr
Pensacola, FL 32514
http://www.nnsdo.org

National Organization for Associate Degree Nursing
11250 Roger Bacon Dr, Suite 8
Reston, VA 11250
http://www.noadn.org

National Student Nurses' Association
455 Main St, Suite 606
Brooklyn, NY 11202
http://www.nsna.org

Nurses Christian Fellowship
Box 7895
Madison, WI 53707-7895
http://www.nfc-jcn.org

Oncology Nursing Society
125 Enterprise Dr
Pittsburgh, PA 15275
http://www.ons.org

Philippine Nurses Association of America, Inc
20127 Avenida Pamplona
Cerritos, CA 90703
http://www.pnaa03.org

Respiratory Nursing Society
7794 Grow Dr
Pensacola, FL 32514-7072

Sigma Theta Tau International Honor Society of Nursing
550 W North St
Indianapolis, IN 46202
http://www.nursing-society.org

Society for Vascular Nursing
7794 Grow Dr
Pensacola, FL 32414

Society of Gastroenterology Nurses and Associates, Inc.
401 North Michigan Ave
Chicago, IL 60611-4267
http://www.sgna.org

Society of Otorhinolaryngology and Head-Neck Nurses, Inc.
116 Canal St
New Smyrna Beach, FL 32168
http://www.sohnnurse.com

Society of Urologic Nurses and Associates
E Holly Ave, Box 56
Pitman, NJ 08071-0056
http://www.suna.org

Transcultural Nursing Society
36600 Schoolcraft Rd
Livonia, MI 48150-1173
http://www.tcns.org

Visiting Nurse Associations of America
99 Summer St, Suite 1700
Boston, MA 02110
http://www.vnaa.org

Wound, Ostomy and Continence Nurses Society
4700 W Lake Ave
Glenview, IL 60025
http://www.wocn.org

U.S. State and Territorial Boards of Nursing

Alabama Board of Nursing
770 Washington Ave
RSA Plaza, Suite 250
Montgomery, AL 36130-3900
http://www.abn.state.al.us

Alaska Board of Nursing
Dept. of Comm. & Econ. Development
Div. of Occupational Licensing
3601 C St, Suite 722
Anchorage, AK 99503
http://www.dced.state.ak.us/occ/pnur.htm

American Samoa Health Services
Regulatory Board
LBJ Tropical Medical Center
Pago Pago, AS 96799

Arizona State Board of Nursing
1651 E Morten Ave, Suite 210
Phoenix, AZ 85020
http://www.azboardof nursing.org

Arkansas State Board of Nursing
University Tower Building
1123 S University, Suite 800
Little Rock, AR 72204-1619
http://www.state.ar.us/nurse

California Board of Registered Nursing
400 R St, Suite 4030
Sacramento, CA 95814
http://www.rn.ca.gov

Colorado Board of Nursing
1560 Broadway, Suite 880
Denver, CO 80202
http://www.dora.state.co.us/nursing

Connecticut Board of Examiners for Nursing
Dept. of Public Health
410 Capitol Ave, MS# 13PHO
Hartford, CT 06134-0328
http://www.state.ct.us/dph

Delaware Board of Nursing
861 Silver Lake Blvd
Cannon Building, Suite 203
Dover, DE 19904

District of Columbia Board of Nursing
Department of Health
825 N Capitol St, NE, 2nd Floor, Room 2224
Washington, DC 20002

Florida Board of Nursing
4080 Woodcock Dr, Suite 202
Jacksonville, FL 32207
http://www.doh.state.fl.us/mga

Georgia Board of Nursing
237 Coliseum Dr
Macon, GA 31217-3858
http://www.sos.state.ga.us/ebd-rn

Guam Board of Nurse Examiners
1304 East Sunset Blvd
Barrgada, Guam 96913

Hawaii Board of Nursing
Professional & Vocational Licensing Division
PO Box 3469
Honolulu, HI 96801
http://www.state.hi.us/dcca/pvl/areasnurse.html

Idaho Board of Nursing
280 N 8th St, Suite 210
Boise, ID 83720
http://www.state.id.us/ibn/ibnhome.htm

Illinois Department of Professional Regulation
James R. Thompson Center
100 West Randolph, Suite 9-300
Chicago, IL 60601
http://www.dpr.state.il.us

Indiana State Board of Nursing
Health Professions Bureau
402 W Washington St, Room W041
Indianapolis, IN 46204
http://www.state.in.us/hpb/boards/isbn

Iowa Board of Nursing
River Point Business
Park
400 SW 8th St, Suite B
Des Moines, IA 50309-
4685

**Kansas State Board of
Nursing**
Landon State Office
Building
900 SW Jackson,
Suite 551-S
Topeka, KS 66612-1230
http://www.ksbn.org

**Kentucky Board of
Nursing**
312 Whittington Pkwy,
Suite 300
Louisville, KY 40222
http://www.kbn.state.
ky.us

**Louisiana State Board
of Nursing**
3510 N Causeway Blvd,
Suite 501
Metairie, LA 70003
http://www.lsbn.state.
la.us

**Maine State Board of
Nursing**
158 State House Station
Augusta, ME 04333
http://www.state.me.us/
boardofnursing

**Maryland Board of
Nursing**
4140 Patterson Ave
Baltimore, MD 21215
http://www.mbon.org

**Massachusetts Board
of Registration in
Nursing**
Commonwealth of
Massachusetts
239 Causeway St
Boston, MA 02114
http://www.state.ma.us/
reg/boards/rn

**Michigan CIS/Office of
Health Services**
Ottawa Towers North
611 W Ottawa, 4th Floor
Lansing, MI 48933
http://www.cis.state.mi.
us/bhser/genover.htm

**Minnesota Board of
Nursing**
2829 University Ave SE,
Suite 500
Minneapolis, MN 55414
http://www.nursing
board.state.mn.us

**Mississippi Board of
Nursing**
1935 Lakeland Dr,
Suite B
Jackson, MS 39216-5014
http://www.msbn.state.
ms.us

**Missouri State Board
of Nursing**
3605 Missouri Blvd
Jefferson City, MO
65102-0656
http://www.ecodev.state.
mo.us/pr/nursing

**Montana Board of
Nursing**
301 South Park
Helena, MT 59620-0513
http://www.discoveringm
ontana.com/dli/bsd/
license

**Nebraska Health and
Human Services
System**
Dept. of Regulation &
Licensure, Nursing
Section
301 Centennial Mall S
Lincoln, NE 68509-4986
http://www.hhs.state.
ne.us/crl/nursingindex.
htm

**Nevada State Board of
Nursing**
License Certification and
Education
4330 S Valley View Blvd,
Suite 106
Las Vegas, NV 89103
http://www.nursingboard.
state.nv.us

**New Hampshire Board
of Nursing**
78 Regional Dr, Bldg B
Concord, NH 03302
http://www.state.nh.us/
nursing

**New Jersey Board of
Nursing**
124 Halsey St, 6th Floor
Newark, NJ 07101
http://www.state.nj.us/
lps/ca/medical.htm

**New Mexico Board of
Nursing**
4206 Louisiana Blvd NE,
Suite A
Albuquerque, NM 87109
http://www.state.nm.us/
clients/nursing

**New York State Board
of Nursing**
Education Bldg
89 Washington Ave
2nd Floor West Wing
Albany, NY 12234
http://www.nysed.gov/
pro/nurse.htm

**North Carolina Board
of Nursing**
3724 National Dr,
Suite 201
Raleigh, NC 27612
http://www.ncbon.com

**North Dakota Board
of Nursing**
919 S 7th St, Suite 504
Bismarck, ND 58504
http://www.ndbon.org

Northern Mariana Islands
Commonwealth Board of
   Nurse Examiners
PO Box 501458
Saipan, MP 96950

Ohio Board of Nursing
17 South High St,
   Suite 400
Columbus, OH 43215-
   3413
http://www.state.oh.us/
   nur

Oklahoma Board of Nursing
2915 N Classen Blvd,
   Suite 524
Oklahoma City, OK
   73106
http://www.your-
   oklahoma.com/nursing

Oregon State Board of Nursing
800 NE Oregon St,
   Box 25
Suite 465
Portland, OR 97232
http://www.osbn.state.
   or.us

Pennsylvania State Board of Nursing
124 Pine St
Harrisburg, PA 17101
http://www.dos.state.
   pa.us/bpoa/nurbd/
   mainpage.htm

Rhode Island Board of Nurse Registration and Nursing Education
105 Cannon Building
Three Capitol Hill
Providence, RI 02908
http://www.health.state.
   ri.us

South Carolina State Board of Nursing
110 Centerview Dr,
   Suite 202
Columbia, SC 29210
http://www.lir.state.sc.us/
   pol/nursing

South Dakota Board of Nursing
4300 South Louise Ave,
   Suite C-1
Sioux Falls, SD 57106-
   3124
http://www.state.sd.us/
   dcr/nursing

Tennessee State Board of Nursing
426 Fifth Ave North
1st Floor, Cordell Hull
   Building
Nashville, TN 37247

Texas Board of Nurse Examiners
333 Guadalupe,
   Suite 3-460
Austin, TX 78701
http://www.bne.state.
   tx.us

Utah State Board of Nursing
Heber M. Wells Bldg,
   4th Floor
160 East 300 South
Salt Lake City, UT
   84111
http://www.commerce.
   state.ut.us

Vermont State Board of Nursing
109 State St
Montpelier, VT 05609-
   1101
http://www.vt
   professionals.org/
   nurses

Virginia Board of Nursing
6606 W. Broad St,
   4th Floor
Richmond, VA 23230
http://www.dhp.state.
   va.us

Washington State Nursing Care Quality Assurance Commission
Department of Health
1300 Quince St SE
Olympia, WA 98504-7846
http://www.doh.wa.gov/
   nursing

West Virginia Board of Examiners for Registered Professional Nurses
101 Dee Dr
Charleston, WV 25311
http://www.state.wv.us/
   nurses/rn

Wisconsin Department of Regulation and Licensing
1400 E Washington Ave
Madison, WI 53708
http://www.drl.state.
   wi.us

Wyoming State Board of Nursing
2020 Carey Ave,
   Suite 110
Cheyenne, WY 82002
http://www.nursing.
   state.wy.us

Resources for NCLEX®
Review Available from
Mosby/Elsevier

For more information on these products and others, please visit our website at *http://www.elsevier.com.*

Mosby's Assesstest: A Practice Exam for RN Licensure, 2006 Unsecured

Dolores F. Saxton, Phyllis K. Pelikan, Judith S. Green, and
    Patricia M. Nugent

Mosby's Assesstest is a practice test composed of 265 questions that reflect the stand-alone format and distribution of content consistent with the latest NCLEX-RN® test plan. Performance is evaluated in categories on client needs, nursing process, clinical area, and focus of care. After taking the exam, students receive a list of questions answered incorrectly as well as a booklet detailing the correct answers, question classifications, and rationales for all answer options.
ISBN: 032303103X

Mosby's Comprehensive Review of Nursing for the NCLEX-RN® Examination, 18th edition

Dolores F. Saxton, Patricia M. Nugent, and Phyllis K.
    Pelikan

This popular review book provides 2490 practice questions to help students prepare for the NCLEX-RN® exam. Its unique coding of questions helps students evaluate performance according to the most recent NCLEX® test plan. A CD-ROM with 1710 additional questions that will provide students with practice on the computer is included.
ISBN: 0323039014

Mosby's Comprehensive Review of Nursing for Review of Nursing for the NCLEX-RN® Examination CD-ROM, 2.0

Dolores F. Saxton, Patrician M. Nugent, and Phyllis K. Pelikan

This CD-ROM offers a thorough outline review of medical-surgical, pediatric, maternity/women's health, and mental health nursing to provide students with a refresher on key nursing content. The content and test questions are also linked with an easy-to-use search function that allows users to move around chapters and between questions.
ISBN: 0323016022

Mosby's Review Cards for the NCLEX-RN® Examination, 2nd edition

Martin S. Manno

These flash cards provide a convenient and portable way for students to study for the NCLEX-RN® examination. This boxed set of review cards contains 1221 NCLEX®-style questions, which include the new alternate item formats. The practice questions, which are organized by clinical area and body system, appear on the front of each card. The reverse side features each question's answer, rationale, cognitive level, nursing process step, and NCLEX® test plan category.
ISBN: 0323040136

Mosby's Review Questions for the NCLEX-RN® Examination, 5th edition

Dolores F. Saxton, Patricia M. Nugent, Phyllis K. Pelikan, and Judith S. Green

This book provides students with more than 3480 practice test questions in both the pencil-and-paper and electronic testing modes. The questions are presented in four distinct formats to meet the needs of students with different study styles and learning needs. Questions in the clinical chapters are grouped by categories or concern; quizzes at the end of each chapter integrate the clinical content; two comprehensive exams parallel the latest NCLEX-RN® test plan; and a CD-ROM with 1220 test questions not duplicated in the book is also included.
ISBN: 0323024688

Mosby's Review Series: Mental Health Nursing

Paulette D. Rollant and Denise B. Deppoliti

Mosby's Review Series provides a comprehensive overview of core nursing content. Designed as a review or clinical resource during undergraduate coursework or in preparation for the NCLEX-RN® exam, these books present essential content in concise outline format. Each book comprises four elements: introductory material, content review, questions and answers, and a comprehensive exam that is also included on disk (both IBM and Macintosh).

ISBN: 0815172478

Mosby's Online Computer Adaptive Test (CAT) for the NCLEX-RN®
Examination, 2nd edition

Dolores F. Saxton, Phyllis K. Pelikan, and Judith S. Green

Mosby's Online CAT for the NCLEX-RN® Examination provides a realistic simulation of the NCLEX-RN® computer adaptive exam and gives instant feedback on test performance. Analysis includes a snapshot of strengths and weaknesses in client needs, nursing behavior, and clinicals. It also gives a reliable "prediction" of success on the NCLEX-RN® exam based on a comparison of individual test performance against a national norm group.

ISBN: 0323028667

Saunders Comprehensive Review for the NCLEX-RN® Examination,
3rd edition, Full Color Reprint

Linda Anne Silvestri

This book and its accompanying CD-ROM provide students with 4000 practice questions. All questions include comprehensive rationales and test-taking strategies. The book covers all the nursing content tested on the NCLEX-RN® exam and also offers chapters on preparation for the NCLEX-RN® exam from a student's perspective. The CD-ROM contains all 1800 multiple choice questions from the book, plus more than 2200 additional practice questions not found in the text.

ISBN: 1416031995

Saunders Computerized Review for the NCLEX-RN® Examination, 2nd edition

Linda Anne Silvestri

This computer-based review tool is specifically designed to help students determine their readiness for the new NCLEX-RN® exam. It generates practice exams from a bank of 2000 questions coded according to content area and category of client needs. Once a student has taken an exam in the test or quiz mode, the CD provides an immediate, detailed analysis of performance. In the review mode, students are given answers that include comprehensive rationales, test-taking strategies, question categories, and references.
ISBN: 0721692370

Saunders Online Review Course for the NCLEX-RN® Examination (offered in 4-, 8-, and 16-week versions)

Linda Anne Silvestri

Saunders Online Review Course for the NCLEX-RN® Examination offers a comprehensive review of core nursing areas and more than 2000 review questions that will assess strengths and weaknesses, focus study time, and increase confidence. A diagnostic pre-test identifies strengths and weaknesses and maps the individual student's course of study. Interactive lessons including animations, video clips, case studies, and mini quizzes and assessments highlight key concepts and reinforce learning.

Saunders Q & A Review for the NCLEX-RN® Examination, 3rd edition

Linda Anne Silvestri

This book/CD-ROM review package is designed to provide students with a total of 5010 NCLEX-RN® exam practice questions. Each practice question provides a complete rationale, test-taking strategy, level of cognitive ability, and text reference. Students also gain valuable practice with alternate item format questions including fill-in-the-blank, multiple response, prioritization, and questions accompanied by a chart, figure, or exhibit. The CD-ROM contains all 1810

practice questions from the book, plus 3200 additional practice questions.
ISBN: 0721603521

Saunders Strategies for Success for the NCLEX-RN® Examination

Linda Anne Silvestri

This text is a critical component of the *Saunders Pyramid to Success* review products for the NCLEX-RN® examination. Whether this is the first or last review product purchased, this book will help students feel well prepared and confident as they prepare for the boards or any exam throughout the nursing curriculum. This book includes test-taking strategies for specific question types including true-false response, prioritization, communication, pharmacology, leadership, and delegation questions. A two-color design, open layout, and casual writing style make this book especially appealing to students. This book would be a great companion to any of the review and testing products currently on the market.
ISBN: 141600095X

Mosby's RNtertainment: An *NCLEX* Review Board Game

Karen Trafton

Mosby's RNtertainment: An NCLEX Review Board Game is a revolutionary game designed as a review tool for nursing students preparing for the NCLEX® exam or for practicing nurses who want to reinforce and sharpen their nursing knowledge. It presents clinical questions and scenarios in all the major nursing categories while providing a fun, humorous, and innovative way to study. Perfect for study groups and gift giving, this game includes a colorful game board, unique die, game pieces, and color-coded category cards that are divided into the four main areas of *Medication, Disease Process/Anatomy & Physiology, Diagnostic Testing*, and *Patient Care*. Two wild card categories titled *Healthy Rewards* and *Code Black and Blue* also incorporate humorous patient scenarios into the game to test the will and ability of a nurse to "handle it all." The object of the game is to travel from start to finish by correctly answering nursing related questions while navigating through the situations randomly faced in the *Healthy Rewards* and *Code Black and Blue* cards.

ISBN: 0323044808

Index

A

Abbreviations, note-taking and, 80
Ability, lack of, failure caused by, 99
Absenteeism, failure caused by, 99
Academic conduct, code of, 177-179
Acronyms, e-mail and use of, 141
Addiction, 7
Address book, for websites, 141
Admission nurse, 4
Adult care center, nurse in, 5
Advance directive, 174
Advanced degree, nursing school
    instructors with, 50, 52
Advisor, 98
Agency for Healthcare Research and
    Quality, website of, 144
Aggressiveness, success or failure
    and, 73-74
AHRQ. *See* Agency for Healthcare
    Research and Quality
Alcohol, avoidance of
  healthy lifestyle and, 118
  nursing student code of conduct
    and, 178
Alta Vista, 141
Alzheimer's disease, 7
Ambiguity, tolerance of, 127
American Cancer Society, website
    of, 144
American Diabetes Association,
    website of, 144
American Hearth Association,
    website of, 144
American Hospital Association,
    patient's bill of rights from,
    171-175
American Nurses Association, 35
  code of ethics from, 175-176
  principles of telehealth from,
    147-149

Page numbers followed by *f* indicate
figures; *t*, tables; *b*, boxes.

ANA. *See* American Nurses
    Association
Anthropologist, nurse as, 8
Anxiety
  clinical skills and, 166, 167
  control of, 132
  oral presentation as cause of, 132
  procrastination as cause of, 105
  test, 87, 88
Armed forces, nursing scholarships
    from, 34-35
Assertiveness
  success or failure and, 74-75
  training for, 75
Associate degree, 27, 28, 31
Attendance, importance of, 57
Attitude
  assertiveness and, 74-75
  nonjudgmental, nurse's need for,
    126-127
  positive, for mature student, 154
  positive or negative, 51
  reading comprehension and, 83
  success and, 73-75
  toward grades, 161-162
Audience
  oral presentation and, 129, 131
  sensitivity to, 132
Audiovisual aid, oral presentation
    with, 133
Author, nurse as, 8

B

Baccalaureate degree, 27, 30
Bachelor's degree, nursing
    instructors with, 51
Balance, healthy lifestyle and, 118
Bedside nurse, 4
Behavior
  code for, 40
  self-defeating, failure caused by,
    99
Bibliography, format for, 136

Bill of rights, patient, 171-175
Billing information, patient's right
    to, 174-175
Boards of nursing, list of, 219-221
Body language, 188-189
Bookmark, for websites, 141
Buckley Amendment, 180
Buddy system, 109-115
Budgeting, importance of, 57
Busywork, avoidance of, 61

C

Caffeine, reduction of, healthy
    lifestyle and, 118
Camp nurse, 5
Canadian nurses, list of associations
    for, 213-214
Canadian Nurses Association, 35
Canadian Nursing Students
    Association, 115
Cardiac nurse, 5
Career guide, 22-24
Careerist syndrome, 121
Case manager, nurse as, 7
CDC. *See* Centers for Disease
    Control and Prevention
Centers for Disease Control and
    Prevention, 6
Change, failure as signal for, 97
Checklist, for nursing success, 18
Chemotherapy, nurse as expert in,
    5
Child care, mature student and,
    158-159
Children, impact of nursing school
    on, 158
Classroom, Internet access in, 140
Clinic, nurse in, 4
Clinical conduct, code of, 177-179
Clinical guidelines, telehealth and,
    148
Clinical nurse specialist, 7
Clinical skills, mastery of, 166-169
Clinical specialist, nurse as, 30
Clinical trials project manager, 6
Code of Academic and Clinical
    Conduct, 177-179
Code of conduct, telehealth and, 147
Code of ethics, American Nurses
    Association and, 175-176
Commitment, lack of, failure caused
    by, 98
Communication, nonverbal, 189
Community, nurse's commitment to,
    176
Competition, in nursing education,
    11
Comprehension, reading skills and,
    83

Computer
    Internet access with, 139
    laptop, 139
Concentration, nursing student's
    need for, 58
Confidence, master of clinical skills
    and, 167-169
Confidentiality
    patient, nursing student code of
        conduct and, 177
    patient's right to, 174
    telehealth and, 148, 149
Consultant, nurse as, 6, 8, 30
Contingency plans, mature student's
    need for, 160
Cooperation, in nursing education, 11
Cost, of nursing education, 33-37
Counseling, 109
Course requirements, nursing
    education and, 40
Courtesy, importance of, 188
Crisis hotline, 7
Critical care nurse, 4
Cruise ship nurse, 6
Curriculum, nursing education and,
    40-41
Cyber cafe, Internet access at, 139
Cyberspace, wasting time in, 142

D

Daily planner, 57
Decision-making, patient's rights
    and, 172
Deferred income, 33-34
Depression
    causes of, 119
    group activity as counter to, 112
Detours, avoidance of, 65-69
Dialysis nurse, 5
Diary, written, 118-119
Dictionary, 59
Differences, tolerance of, 127
Dignity, patient, 161
Diploma program, 27, 28, 31
Director, nurse as, 30
Disappointment, failure and, 100-101
Distractions, avoidance of, 60
Diversions, avoidance of, 66
Doctorate, nursing instructors with,
    51
Doctor's office, nurse in, 4
Documentation
    importance of, 182
    telehealth and, 148
Domain name, e-mail access and, 141
Dress code, 40
Drug companies
    websites produced by, 143
Drug handbook, 59

E

E-mail, 140
Editor, nurse as, 8
Education, cost of, 33-37
Educator, nurse as, 4, 7
Effectiveness, nursing student's
    need for, 55
Efficiency, nursing student's need
    for, 55
Effort, talent and, 163
80/20 principle, 56-57
Electives, 121-123
Employee-assistance program, nurse
    working in, 7
Employment
    conditions of, 176
    fringe benefits in, 3, 22-24
    part-time, in health care industry,
        69
    salary level of, 3, 24, 179
Environment, safe, patient's right to,
    172
Equipment, for nursing student, 58
Equipment companies
    websites produced by, 143
Essay test questions, 93
Ethicist, nurse as, 8
Ethics, nursing student code of
        conduct and, 178
Exam. *See* Tests and testing
Exercise, healthy lifestyle and, 118
Eye contact, 188-189

F

Faculty
    joint appointments for, 185
    work load of, 72-73
Failure
    definition of, 97
    disappointment of others and,
        100-101
    reasons for, 98-101
Family
    nurse's commitment to, 176
    support from, 156-158
    time for, 160
Federal Trade Commission, 142-143
Filing system, nursing student's
    need for, 59
Fill-in-the-blank test questions, 92
Financial aid
    for nursing education, 34-36
    sources of, 205-208
First impressions, 187-188
Flexibility, nurse's need for, 126
Flight-for-life nurse, 4
Food and Drug Administration,
    website of, 144

Footnotes, format for, 136
Fringe benefits, 22-24
FTC. *See* Federal Trade Commission

G

Genetic counseling, nurse as expert
    in, 5
Gerontology nurse, 5
Goals
    importance of, 66-68
    long-term, 66
    nursing student's need for, 59-60
    realistic, 69
Google, 141, 143
Grades
    attitude toward, 161-162
    poor, procrastination as cause of,
        105
Graduation, as long-term goal, 66-68
Grants, 34-35
Group, nurse's commitment to, 176
Group activity, 109, 110
    benefits of, 111-112
Guidance counselor, 98
Guidelines, clinical, telehealth and,
    148
Guilt, procrastination as cause of,
    105

H

Handouts, oral presentation with,
    133
Hate groups, on Internet, 145
Head nurse, 30
Health, preventive maintenance for,
    117-119
Health and fitness industry, nurse
    working in, 7
Health care
    legal issues in, 181
    patient goals in, 173
    patient's right to, 171-175
Health care power of attorney,
    173-174
Health information, websites for,
    143, 144
Health on the Net Foundation,
    website of, 144
Health screening, 6
HealthAtoZ.com, website of, 144
Higher education agencies, 205-208
Homesickness, 109
Hospital
    benefits offered by, 22-24
    nursing in, 4, 7
    part-time job in, 69
    patient's rights and, 172-175
    percentage of nurses working in,
        16

Hospital *(Continued)*
  student nurse orientation in,
      186-187
Hospital care, patient's right to, 172
Housework, 155-156
Humor, healthy lifestyle and, 118
Husband, support from, 155-158

I

Illness, failure caused by, 98
Indecision, avoidance of, 62
Indian Health Service, 6
Infection control nurse, 4
Inferiority, sense of, 74
Information
  integrity of
      in health care systems, 148
  patient's right to, 172-173
  retention of, 78
Informed consent, 180-181
  telehealth and, 149
Inner voice, 79
Instructor
  nurse as, 30
  philosophy of, 49, 50
  in school of nursing, 49-53
  working with, 72-73
Insurance, malpractice, 181
Insurance claim, 174
Insurance company, nurse as
      employee of, 6
Internet, 139-149. *See also* Websites
  abuse of, 142, 143
  access to, 139
  in classroom, 140
  search engines for, 141-142
  wireless access to, 140
Internet provider, 139
Investigator, nurse as, 6

J

Job security, 3
Journals
  personal, 118-119
  web access to, 145
Junk mail, 142

L

Language, medical, 81
Lawsuit, nurse as defendant in, 181
Laziness, failure caused by, 98
Learning
  grades and, 161-162
  listening and, 79-81
Legal nurse consultant, 6
Librarian
  nursing student's use of, 61
  research help from, 134
Library, Internet access at, 139

Library of Medicine, website of, 144
Licensure, professional, telehealth
      and, 147, 148
Lifelong learning, nursing student
      code of conduct and, 178
Listening, importance of, 79-81
Lists, nursing student's need for,
      60-61
Litigation, avoidance of, 181
Living will, 174
Loans, 34-35
  sources of, 205-208
Loneliness, group activity to
      counter, 110
Long-term memory, 77, 84

M

Malpractice insurance, 181
Manager, nurse as, 4
Marriage, mature student and,
      154-155
Master's degree, nursing instructors
      with, 51
Matching item test questions, 92
Mathematical test questions, 92
Mature student, 153-163
Mayo Clinic, website of, 144
Medical/nursing dictionary, 59
Medical reference books, 59
Medical-surgical nurse, 5
MEDLINE plus, website of, 144
Medscape, website of, 144
Memory
  exercises for, 78-79
  long-term, 77, 84
  short-term, 77
Mentoring, nursing student code of
      conduct and, 178
Merck Medical Manual, 59
Midlife, returning to school at, 153
Midwife, nurse as, 5
Military
  nurse working in, 7
  nursing scholarships from, 34-35
Minnesota Multiphasic Personality
      Inventory, 51
Missionary, nurse as, 6
MMPI. *See* Minnesota Multiphasic
      Personality Inventory
Mnemonics, memory skills and, 78-79
Modem, Internet access with, 139
Moderation, healthy lifestyle and,
      118
Morale, group activity and, 114
Multiple-choice test questions, 91

N

National Institutes of Health, 6
  website of, 144

National League for Nursing, 35
National Library of Medicine,
     website of, 144
National Student Nurses
     Association, 35, 43, 115
  code of academic and clinical
     conduct from, 177-179
NCLEX review, resources for,
     223-228
Neonatal intensive care unit, nurse
     in, 5
Netiquette, 141
Networking, study group for, 115
Neuroscience nurse, 4
Newborn nursery, nurse in, 5
NICU. *See* Neonatal intensive care
     unit
NIH. *See* National Institutes of
     Health
Nonverbal communication, 189
Note-taking
  abbreviations used in, 80
  skills for, 80-81
  from textbooks, 83
Notice of Privacy Practices, 174
Nurse
  attitudes of, 126-127
  Canadian, list of associations for,
     213-214
  code of ethics for, 175-176
  as consultant, 6
  demand for, 15-16
  education for, 27-31
  list of state associations for,
     209-211
  nonjudgmental attitude of, 126
  personal *versus* professional
     modes of, 161
  registered, 21-24
     education for, 27-31
     licensure of, 28
  responsibility of, for conduct,
     151
  retention of, 23
  salary for, 3, 24
  shortages of, 16
  specialty, organizations for,
     215-218
  success tips for, 43-47
  successful, 13-14
  types of, 3-8
Nurse anesthetist, 4
Nurse anthropologist, 8
Nurse associations, list of, 209-211
Nurse attorney, 6, 181-182
Nurse ethicist, 8
Nurse midwife, 5
Nurse practitioner, 7, 30
Nurse sociologist, 8

Nursing
  advancement of, 176
  alternatives in, 125
  boards of, 219-221
  career guide for, 22-24
  checklist for success in, 18
  clinical skills in, 166
  code of ethics for, 175-176
  degrees in, 27-31
  demand in, 15-16
  description of, 3-8, 14-17
  education in, 27-31
  fringe benefits in, 3, 22-24
  legal issues in, 181
  list of Canadian associations for,
     23-214
  list of state associations of,
     209-211
  pace of change in, 14-15
  prefixes used in, 199-204
  responsible conduct in, 151
  salary in, 3, 24
  specialty, organizations for,
     215-218
  state and territorial boards of,
     219-221
  state board examination for, 192-193
  success in, 13-14
  suffixes used in, 199-204
  telehealth impact on, 146-149
  types of, 3-8
Nursing education, 11
  cost of, 33-37
  elective courses in, 121-123
  final year of, 191-193
  financial aid for, 34-36
  grades in, 161-162
  mastering skills in, 166
  nursing service and, 186
  rules and regulations in, 39-41
  standardization in, 51
  success tips for, 43-47
  teachers in, 49-53
Nursing faculty, 49-53
Nursing home
  nurse in, 5
  nursing in, 5
Nursing program, 27
  cost of, 33-37
Nursing service, nursing education
     and, 186
Nursing skills, mastery of, 166,
     167-169
Nursing skills lab, 166
Nursing student
  assertiveness in, 74-75
  attitudes of, 73-75
  code of academic and clinical
     conduct for, 177-179

Nursing student *(Continued)*
  elective courses for, 121-123
  failure of, 97-101
  final year of education of, 191-193
  freshman, homesickness in, 109
  goal-oriented, 68, 69
  goals of, 59-60, 66-68
  healthy lifestyle for, 117-119
  hospital orientation for, 186-187
  loneliness in, 110
  mature, 153-163
  part-time job and, 69
  personal *versus* professional
      modes of, 161
  positive or negative attitude of, 51
  priorities of, 66-68
  problem solving skills for, 71-73
  respect for, 179
  rights of, 180
  study group for, 111-115
  support from spouse for, 155-158
  time management for, 57-63
Nursing textbooks, 58-59, 81, 83

O

Occupational health nurse, 7
Oncology, nurse in, 5
Operating room, nurse in, 4
Orientation program, 109
Orthopedic nurse, 5
Outline, for writing assignment, 134,
    135
Outside activities, failure caused by,
    100

P

Palliative care nurse, 5
Panic, test anxiety and, 88
Paperwork, importance of, 182
Paraphrasing, information retention
    and, 78
Parish nurse, 6
Parkinson's Law, 61
Patient
  bill of rights for, 171-175
  nurse's commitment to, 176
  respect for, 188
  rights of, 171-174, 175
  safe environment for, 172
Patient advocate, nurse as, 4
Patient care, nurse role in, 17
Patient care partnership, 171-175
Patient Care Partnership:
    Understanding Expectations,
    Rights and Responsibilities,
    175
PDA. *See* Personal digital assistant
Peace Corps, 6
Pediatric nurse, 5

Personal digital assistant, 57, 139
Personal growth, 176
Personal identification number, 142
Petition, solving a problem with, 73
Photocopying, nursing student's use
    of, 63
PIN. *See* Personal identification
    number
Planning, importance of, 67-68
Pornography, on Internet, 145
Postanesthesia nurse, 4
Power of attorney, health care,
    173-174
Prefixes
  common, in nursing, 199-204
  medical language and, 81
Prenatal care, nurse as expert in, 5
Presentation, oral
  content of, 130
  organization of, 129-130
Prime time, use of, 62
Priorities
  importance of, 66-68
  nursing student's need for, 56-57,
      60
Prison, nurse working in, 7
Privacy
  mature student's need for, 158
  patient, 161
  patient's right to, 174
Problem solving, 71-73
Procrastination
  avoidance of, 60
  overcoming, 105-106
  psychology of, 104
Productivity, group activity and
    increase in, 112
Profession, dress and behavior codes
    for, 40
Professional growth, 176
  nursing student code of conduct
      and, 178
Professional journals, web access to,
    145
Professional standards, telehealth
    and, 147
Professionalism, student nurse and,
    187
Psychiatric nursing, 125
Psychology, learning and, 73-74
Public health nurse, 5, 30

Q

Quality assurance, nurse and, 4
Questionnaire, for nursing success,
    18

R

Radiation, nurse as expert in, 5

Reading, 81-84
  amount of, in nursing school, 82
  comprehension of, 83
  speed of, 83
Reading level, in nursing textbooks,
    82, 83
Reading skills, 82
  nursing student's need for, 55
Reference books, 59
Registered nurse, 21-24
  education for, 27-31
  licensure of, 28
Rehabilitation, nurse in, 4
Rehearsal, for oral presentation,
    130-131
Research
  on telehealth, 149
  for writing assignment, 134-135
Research nurse, 6
Researcher, nurse as, 4, 30
Resources, for NCLEX review,
    223-228
Respect
  for nurse, 179
  for nursing student, 179
Responsibility
  health care professional, patient's
    rights and, 171-175
  nurse's, 151
  nursing student code of conduct
    and, 178
Rest, healthy lifestyle and, 118
Rest-and-relaxation, 63
Root word, medical language and, 81
Rules and regulations, nursing
    schools and, 39-41
Rumination, depression and, 119

S

Safety
  in hospital environment, 172
  nursing student code of conduct
    and, 178
  patient's rights for, 172
  telehealth and, 149
Salary, level of, 3, 24, 179
Sales representative, nurse as, 8
SANE. See Sexual Assault Nurse
    Examiner
Schedule, nursing, 3
Scholarships, 34-35
  sources of, 205-208
School nurse, 6
School of nursing, 7
  enrollment levels in, 15-16
  faculty in, 49-53
  Internet access at, 139
  rules and regulations in, 39-41
  teachers in, 49-53

Scrub nurse, 4
Self-actualization, 117
Self-confidence, 105
Self-esteem, 74, 105
Self-medication, telehealth and, 146
Sense of humor, healthy lifestyle
    and, 118
Sequencing, 159
Sexual Assault Nurse Examiner, 6
Short-term memory, 77
Shorthand, note-taking and, 80
Sleep, nursing student's need for, 63
Social Security number, Internet use
    and, 142
Sociologist, nurse as, 8
Software, Internet access with, 139
Spam, e-mail and, 142
Speaking skills, 129-133
  improvement in, 131
Specialist, nurse as, 4
Specialization, nursing school
    instructors and, 50
Speech, preparation for, 129-133
Spell checker, 135-136
  e-mail and, 141
Spelling, spell checker correction of,
    135-136
Spouse, support from, 155, 156-158
Standardization, nursing education
    requirements and, 51
State board examination, 28, 94-95,
    192-193
State boards of nursing, 219-221
State higher education agencies,
    205-208
Street smarts, 185-189
Stress
  avoidance of, healthy lifestyle and,
    118
  mature student and, 160
Stress management, 117
Stress management specialist, nurse
    as, 7
Student nurse. See Nursing student
Study group, 89, 111-115
  ground rules for, 113-115
  successful, 113-114
Study habits, 103-107
  poor, failure caused by, 99-100
Study skills, poor, failure caused by,
    99-100
Study time, mature student's need
    for, 158
Success, tips for, 43-47
Suffixes
  common, in nursing, 199-204
  medical language and, 81
Suicide prevention, 7
Supervisor, nurse as, 4

Superwoman complex, 155, 159-160
Support group, 111, 115
Surgical nurse, 4
Survival tips, for nursing education,
  43-47
Symbols, note-taking and, 80

T

Talent, hard work and, 163
Tape recorder, rehearsal for oral
  presentation with, 130-131
Teacher
  nurse as, 30
  philosophy of, 49, 50
  in school of nursing, 49-53
  working with, 72-73
Teaching, nurse in, 7
Telehealth, 146-149
Telenursing, 146
Telepatient, 146-147
"Ten Basic Rights for Nurses in the
  Health Professions," 179-180
Term paper, 103
  on Internet, 145
  topic for, 134
Territorial boards of nursing, 219-221
Test anxiety, 87, 88
Tests and testing
  essay questions on, 93
  fill-in-the-blank, 92
  frequency of, 89
  length of, 90
  matching items, 92
  mathematical items, 92
  multiple-choice, 91
  NCLEX review, resources for,
    223-228
  preparation for, 88-94
  short answer, 92
  state board exam, 94-95
  studying for, 89
  true-false, 91-92
  types of questions on, 90-94
Textbooks, 58-59
  note-taking from, 83
  reading level in, 81
Thesaurus, 59
Time management, 57-63
Title page, importance of, 136
"To do" list, 65
  nursing student's need for, 58
Tobacco, avoidance of, healthy
  lifestyle and, 118
Tolerance, nurse's need for, 126
Transplant team, nurse on, 4-5
Transport nurse, 4
Trauma nurse, 4
Traveling nurse agency, 6
Treatment plan, patient's right to, 173

True-false test questions, 91-92
Tuition, for nursing program, 33

U

Urgent care nurse, 4
US Department of Health and
  Human Services, website of,
  144
US National Library of Medicine,
  website of, 144

V

Vacillation, avoidance of, 62
Veterans hospital, nurse in, 7
Video conferencing, health care and,
  146
Visiting nurse, 5
Visualization
  mastery of clinical skills and, 167
  memory skills and, 78
Vitamins, healthy lifestyle and, 118

W

Walk-On-Water Woman, 159-160
Web Crawler, 141
WebMD, website of, 144
Websites. *See also* Internet
  address of, 141
  growth of, 143
  for health information, 143, 144
  for NCLEX review resources, 223
  nursing information at, 16, 34
  producers of, 143
  research for writing assignments
    on, 134
  search engines for, 141-142
Wellness, preventive maintenance
  for, 117-119
WHO. *See* World Health
  Organization
Women, depression in, 119
Word processor, spell checker in, 135
Workload, nurse's, 179
World Health Organization, 6
  website of, 144
World Wide Web, 139-149
  addresses on, 141
  search engines for, 141-142
Writing assignment
  drafts of, 135
  organization of, 133-134
  topic for, 134
Writing skills, 133-135
  nursing student's need for, 55
WWW. *See* World Wide Web

Y

Yahoo, 141